ARRHYTHMIAS AND SUDDEN DEATH IN ATHLETES

Developments in Cardiovascular Medicine

VOLUME 232

Arrhythmias and Sudden Death in Athletes

edited by

A. BAYÉS DE LUNA

Institut Catala Cardiologia-Hosp.,
Sant Pau, Barcelona, Spain

F. FURLANELLO

Istituto Scientifico H.S. Raffaele,
Milan-Rome, Italy

B.J. MARON

Minneapolis Heart Institute Foundation,
Minneapolis, Minnesota, U.S.A.

and

D.P. ZIPES

Krannert Institute of Cardiology,
Indiana University School of Medicine and
the Roudebush Veterans Administration Medical Center,
Indianapolis, Indiana, U.S.A.

KLUWER ACADEMIC PUBLISHERS
DORDRECHT / BOSTON / LONDON

A C.I.P. Catalogue record for this book is available from the Library of Congress.

ISBN 0-7923-6337-X

Published by Kluwer Academic Publishers,
P.O. Box 17, 3300 AA Dordrecht, The Netherlands.

Sold and distributed in North, Central and South America
by Kluwer Academic Publishers,
101 Philip Drive, Norwell, MA 02061, U.S.A.

In all other countries, sold and distributed
by Kluwer Academic Publishers,
P.O. Box 322, 3300 AH Dordrecht, The Netherlands.

Printed on acid-free paper

Printed in the Netherlands.

FOREWORD

Cardiovascular diseases are the most important causes of death in the world today. In adults, the most frequent heart disease is acute myocardial infarction, which can lead to sudden death. To prevent these diseases we need to fight against their main risk factors, which include smoking, lipid disorders, hypertension, diabetes and a sedentary life-style, among others.

It has been demonstrated that physical exercise or sports at any age provide notable benefits and can help to decrease other risk factors and reduce the incidence of cardiovascular diseases. Exercise can be simply walking or cycling. Aerobic exercise contributes to weight loss and also helps to control blood pressure, cholesterol and diabetes. It therefore plays an important role in prevention of heart diseases.

Sports for young people are of great value and advisable not only because they contribute to physical fitness but also because they help in psychological well-being. Young people should be encouraged to include general exercise, and particularly sports, into their daily activities.

The following points however, should be kept in mind:

1. Although winning at a sport is important, this is only so if it is achieved in natural physical conditions and with the correct training. Therefore, it is advisable to keep well away from any type of activity which artificially increases physical performance, that is, drug taking.

2. Sportsmen and women should undergo regular health check-ups, especially from a cardiovascular viewpoint, so as to rule out the danger of presenting severe complications, particularly the rare but dramatic occurrence of sudden death.

This book, edited by Drs. Antonio Bayés de Luna, Francesco Furlanello, Barry Maron and Douglas Zipes, describes the problems related to sudden death in athletes from a scientific viewpoint. Although I am no expert, I believe that this publication covers all aspects related to this subject and the extraordinary challenge it entails. Consequently, it may be particularly useful for physicians and other health care personnel working in the field of sports medicine, as it provides the necessary knowledge for determining when an athlete is at risk of presenting a severe cardiovascular disease, or even sudden death, and what should be done for their prevention.

I would like to congratulate the editors of this book for their excellent contribution to the field, the magnitude of which will allow athletes, both professional and amateur, to participate in sporting activities with a maximum guarantee for their cardiovascular health.

Juan Antonio Samaranch
Marquis de Samaranch
President International Olympic Committee

CONTENTS

CHAPTER 1

SCOPE OF THE PROBLEM OF SUDDEN DEATH IN ATHLETES: DEFINITIONS, EPIDEMIOLOGY AND SOCIOECONOMIC IMPLICATIONS

B.J. Maron
Minneapolis Heart Institute Foundation, Minneapolis, Minnesota, USA

Introduction

Over the past several years, there has been increasing interest and concern in the medical community and among the lay public regarding sudden and unexpected catastrophes in young trained athletes (1) (Fig. 1). The risks associated with participation in organized competitive sports have proved to be diverse, ranging from sudden collapse due to a variety of underlying (and usually unsuspected) cardiovascular diseases (2-11) or from non-penetrating chest impact (12-15).

Although these events are devastating, they are nevertheless uncommon relative to the vast numbers of young athletes participating safely in a wide variety of sporting activities (16). Therefore, it is important that information about athletic field deaths not raise undue anxiety and thereby unnecessarily inhibit sports participation. On the other hand, the sudden deaths of young athletes remains an important medical and societal issue. Uncertainty about the level of risk incurred by apparently healthy young persons participating in competitive sports represents a persistent source of concern for athletes as well as their parents and family, coaches and health care providers. Indeed, it is an important medical responsibility to create an informed public and, to pursue when practical, early detection of those diseases or conditions that may be responsible for catastrophic events in young athletes, as well as to design potentially effective preventive measures.

The news media have to some extent sensationalized these tragedies by routinely making the deaths of young athletes into news events with widespread access to the public domain (Fig. 1). However, this very process has also been instrumental in bringing many issues regarding sudden death in the young to our awareness, and also permitted important retrospective research on this subject (2, 3).

In the present discussion (which excludes considerations related to middle-aged athletes and the many benefits of exercise for the general population) an attempt has been made to place into perspective the cardiovascular risks associated with organized sports competition in order to create a safer sports environment for young athletes.

1

A. Bayés de Luna et al. (eds.), Arrhythmias and Sudden Death in Athletes, 1–10.
© 2000 *Kluwer Academic Publishers. Printed in the Netherlands.*

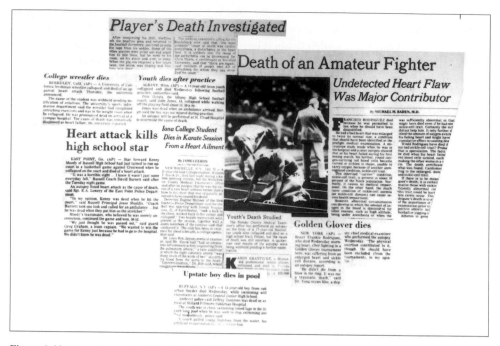

Figure 1. News media reports of sudden death in athletes.

Definition

A competitive athlete is defined as one who participates in an organized team or individual sport that requires regular competition against others as a central component, places a high premium on excellence and achievement, and requires vigorous and intense training in a systematic fashion (17). It should also be emphasized that many individuals participate in "recreational" sports in a truly competitive fashion.

Epidemiological Profile of Sudden Death in Athletes

PREVALENCE

Although generally acknowledged to be very uncommon, the precise frequency with which sudden and unexpected cardiovascular deaths occur in young athletes during organized competitive sports is not known with certainty. Indeed, there are a number of practical obstacles to the assembly of such data. Prevalence estimates of sudden death that rely on reporting from individual schools and institutions, or on media accounts (2, 3), probably underestimate the occurrence of these events throughout large geographic areas, such as the United States. To date, the best available figures based on national or state populations suggest that, despite the broad participation in organized sports, sudden deaths due to cardiovascular disease in high school or college-aged athletes are rare, occurring in about 1:200,000 (16) to 1:300,000 (3) individuals per academic year and (about 1:70,000 for a given athlete over a 3-year high school career) (16). In comparison, somewhat higher rates for sudden death related to exercise have been reported for apparently healthy males (18), joggers (19, 20) or marathon racers (21) (*i.e.*, about 1:15,000 to 1:50,000 per year).

Taken together such estimates suggest that the intense and persistent public interest in these devastating events is perhaps disproportionate to their overall numerical impact on society. Nevertheless, the emotional, medical, and societal consequences of these events in young people remain high. To most of the lay public and medical community the competitive athlete symbolizes the healthiest segment of our society and the unexpected collapse of such young people is a powerful event that inevitably strikes to the core of our sensibilities (1). For these reasons, and despite its low event rate, sudden death in young athletes will continue to represent an important medical issue.

DEMOGRAPHICS
Based primarily on data assembled from a broad-based United States population (2), a profile of young competitive athletes who die suddenly has emerged. Such athletes participated in a large number and variety of sports with the most frequent being basketball and football [about 70% (Fig. 2), probably reflecting the intense physical exertion involved and also the high participation rates in these popular team sports in the United States]. Most athletes are of high school age at the time of death (about 60%); however, other sudden deaths occur in young athletes who have achieved collegiate or even professional levels of competition.

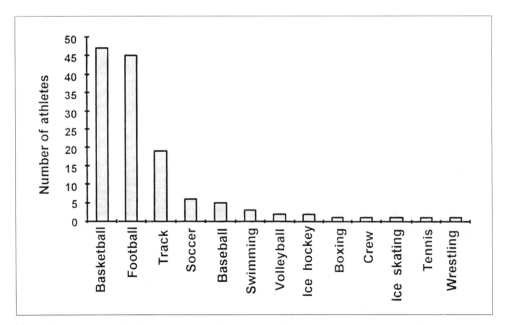

Figure 2. Sports engaged in at the time of sudden death in 134 young competitive athletes. Those competing in track events were either distance runners or sprinters. Reproduced from Maron *et al.* (2) with permission of American Medical Association.

Athletic field deaths show a clear gender predilection with striking male predominance (90%). That only about 10% of these events occur in female athletes (2, 3) may be explained because women: i) participate less commonly in high school and collegiate sports programs than men (by about 2:1) (3); ii) are often exposed to generally less intensive training demands than men; and iii) do not participate in certain sports (such as football) which are associated with a high risk for sudden death.

The vast majority of athletes who incur sudden death have been free of cardiovascular symptoms during their lives and had not been suspected to harbor cardiovascular disease. Sudden collapse usually occurs associated with physical exertion (in 90% of cases), predominantly in the late afternoon and early evening hours corresponding to the peak periods of competition and training, particularly in organized team sports such as football and basketball (Fig. 3) (2). These observations substantiate that, in the presence of certain underlying structural cardiovascular diseases, physical activity represents a trigger and an important precipitating factor for sudden collapse on the athletic field.

This predilection for sudden death late in the day is similar in athletes with hypertrophic cardiomyopathy (HCM) as well as in athletes with other lesions. For athletes with HCM, however, this observation contrasts strikingly with prior findings in patients with HCM (who were *not* competitive athletes) for whom a bimodal pattern of circadian variability over the 24-h day was evident, including a prominent early to mid-morning peak similar to that reported in patients with coronary artery disease (Fig. 3) (22).

RACE

Race also appears to play a role in the demographics of athletic field deaths. Although the majority of reported sudden deaths in competitive athletes are in whites, a substantial proportion (>40%), nevertheless, have been in African-Americans (23, 24). Furthermore, HCM appears to be a common cause of sudden death in African-American male athletes (Fig. 4). This latter observation contrasts sharply with the infrequent reports of African-American patients with HCM in hospital-based tertiary center populations (23, 24). Therefore, HCM is encountered in young African-Americans largely when the disease results in sudden and unexpected death during competitive athletics. The most likely explanation for these findings is disproportionate access to subspecialty medical care and cardiovascular diagnosis on a socioeconomic basis between the African-American and white communities in the United States, making it less likely that young black males will either be identified with HCM or consequently disqualified from competition to reduce their risk for sudden death (in accordance with the recommendations of 26th Bethesda Conference) (17).

Other Risks of the Athletic Field Unrelated to Underlying Cardiovascular Disease

While sudden death in young athletes due to unsuspected and largely congenital heart diseases (2-11) has achieved great visibility, other risks of organized or recreational sports activity leading to cardiovascular collapse have been emphasized more recently. For example, although apparently uncommon, virtually instantaneous cardiac arrest may result from a relatively modest and nonpenetrating blow to the chest – in the *absence* of underlying cardiovascular disease (12-15, 24, 25) or structural injury to the chest wall or heart itself.

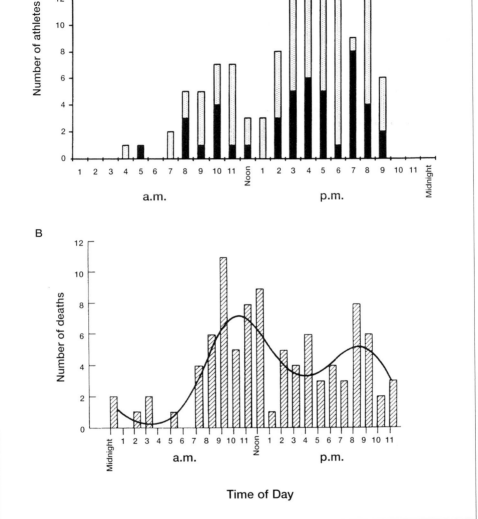

Figure 3. Hourly distribution of sudden cardiac deaths suggesting that intense physical activity acts as a trigger for sudden cardiac death in athletes with underlying structural cardiac disease. A) Histogram showing time of death in 127 competitive athletes either with hypertrophic cardiomyopathy (HCM) (bold portion of bars) or a variety of other predominantly congenital cardiovascular malformations (lighter portions of bars). Time of death was predominantly in the late afternoon and early evening, corresponding largely to the time of training and competition. Reproduced from Maron *et al.* (2) with permission of the American Medical Association. B) In contrast, shown for 94 patients with HCM (who were not competitive athletes), demonstrating a prominent early peak between 7 a.m. and 1 p.m. and a secondary peak in the early evening (most evident between 8 p..m. and 10 p.m.). Reproduced from Maron *et al.* (22) with permission of the J Am Coll Cardiol.

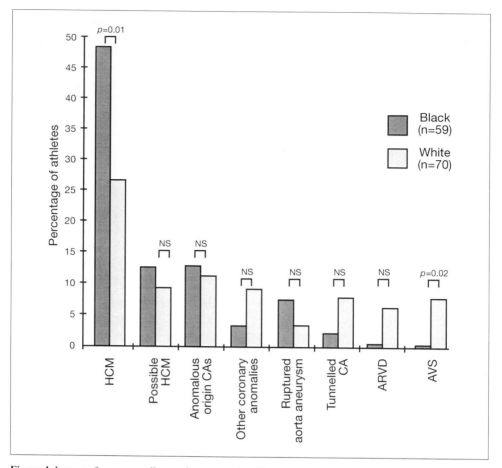

Figure 4. Impact of race on cardiovascular causes of sudden death in competitive athletes. AVS = aortic valve stenosis; CA = coronary anomalies; HCM = hypertrophic cardiomyopathy. Reproduced from Maron *et al.* (23) with permission of the American Medical Association.

In such occurrences, which have been referred to as commotio cordis ("disturbed or agitated heart motion"), blunt chest impact over the anatomic position of the heart is usually produced by a projectile (most commonly a baseball or a hockey puck at close range), or by bodily collision with another athlete. The chest blow is not perceived as unusual for the sporting event, nor necessarily of sufficient magnitude to result in a cat-astrophe. A common scenario during competitive sports is that of a young baseball player struck in the chest (while batting) by a pitched ball thrown from a standard dis-tance. Of note, many of these catastrophes have occurred in purely recreational situa-tions at home or on the playground, with the fatal injuries often produced by family members. A recently developed experimental model in juvenile swine closely simulates the clinical profile of commotio cordis and provides important insights with the respon-sible mechanisms. The model shows that a precordial blow can create devastating elec-trophysiological consequences largely by virtue of its precise timing. When chest impact occurs, with modest force (50 km/h), during a very narrow window of 15-30 ms prior to the T-wave peak, it interferes with the vulnerable phase of repolarization and ventricular fibrillation results instantaneously and reproducibly (14). Furthermore, softer-than-standard safety baseballs reduced the risk for ventricular fibrillation, suggesting that the prevention of sudden death from commotio cordis during certain youth sporting activities may be achieved through the modification of athletic equipment (14).

Commotio cordis events are not uniformly fatal and about 10% of reported victims are known to have survived, usually associated with reasonably prompt cardiopulmonary resuscitation and defibrillation (13, 25). With enhanced public awareness of this syndrome, emergency measures are more likely to be implemented promptly on the athletic field, possibly avoiding many future catastrophes.

It is also evident that relatively modest nonpenetrating chest blows, usually by the high-velocity impact delivered by a soccer ball, are also capable of producing nonfatal acute myocardial infarction in the absence of underlying disease, which may ultimately result in ventricular dysfunction and even aneurysm formation (24). Although the precise mechanism of such events is uncertain, direct compression of an extramural coronary artery could produce spasm or thrombosis, or mechanically disrupt a preexisting atherosclerotic plaque, resulting in myocardial ischemia and infarction.

Preparticipation Screening and Detection of Cardiovascular Abnormalities

Detection of preexisting cardiovascular abnormalities with the potential for significant morbidity or sudden death is an important objective of preparticipation screening (26). In the United States, large-scale athletic screening has traditionally been performed in the context of a history (personal and family) and physical examination. However, the practicality and utility of the screening process is limited by the following: i) the uncommon occurrence (within the general population) of these relevant cardiovascular lesions and the difficulty in clinical identification of some conditions, such as congenital coronary anomalies and arrhythmogenic right ventricular dysplasia; and ii) the large size of the competitive athletic population (perhaps 10 million every year in the United States). Indeed, one retrospective study showed that cardiovascular abnormalities were suspected by standard history and physical examination screening in only 3% of the high school and collegiate athletes who ultimately died suddenly from cardiac disease (2). The rate of detection of cardiovascular lesions is ultimately much higher when suspicion is raised by primary screening (Fig. 5).

An American Heart Association consensus panel (26) has recently supported the principle of preparticipation cardiovascular screening for young competitive athletes on both medical and ethical grounds. The panel recommended a history (personal and family) and physical examination targeted to the cardiovascular lesions known to be responsible for sudden death or disease progression (although imperfect) as the most practical and best available strategy for screening large youthful athletic populations. In addition, the panel offered specific recommendations regarding the composition of the history and physical examination, as well as the selection of examiners.

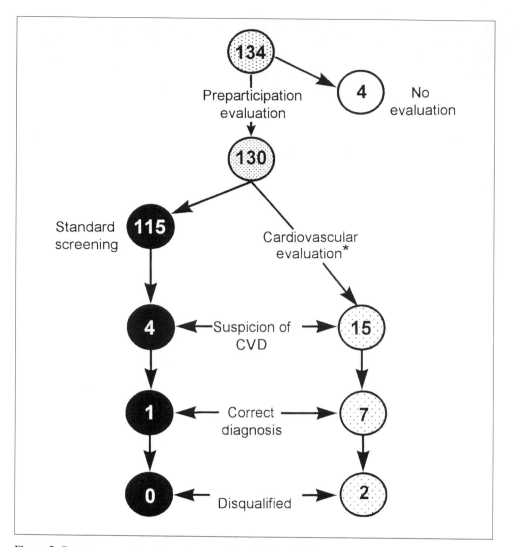

Figure 5. Consequences of cardiovascular screening of high school and college-aged athletes. Flow diagram showing impact of preparticipation medical history and physical examination on the detection of structural cardiovascular disease (and causes of sudden death), as well as subsequent disqualification from competitive athletes. *Cardiovascular evaluation with testing (independent of standard school or institutional preparticipation screening), performed in 15 athletes because of cardiac symptoms, family history of heart disease, heart murmur, or physical findings suggestive of cardiovascular disease. Reproduced from Maron *et al.* (2) with permission of the American Medical Association.

Preparticipation examinations in the United States occur largely at the discretion of the examining physician as customary practice, based on requirements of high schools and colleges. A considerably different, and perhaps the largest screening effort for the detection of cardiovascular abnormalities in athletic populations (routinely involving 12-lead ECGs), has been mandated in Italy since 1982 as part of a national evaluation program for competitive athletes (27). In this unique program, supported financially by the Italian government, all citizens (ages 12-35) who wish to engage in organized sports activities must achieve annual medical clearance from an approved physician stipulating the athlete to be free of abnormalities that could unacceptably increase the risk of sudden death during training or competition. Of note, Italian physicians in the Veneto region of northeastern Italy have recently demonstrated the utility of systematic preparticipation screening in the detection of otherwise unrecognized hypertrophic cardiomyopathy in young competitive athletes primarily by virtue of the 12-lead ECG, in addition to the history and physical examination (28).

While the addition of noninvasive testing (such as echocardiography and/or ECG) to preparticipation screening would enhance the identification of many cardiovascular abnormalities (26, 28), it should be emphasized that no large scale screening effort (even with diagnostic testing), can detect all or even most important lesions or affected athletes (26). Consequently, medical clearance for sports should not promulgate a false sense of security or an unrealistic expectation that the athlete is absolutely free of potentially lethal cardiovascular disease.

References

1. Maron, B.J. *Sudden death in young athletes: Lessons from the Hank Gathers affair.* N Engl J Med 1993, 329: 55-7.
2. Maron, B.J., Shirani, J., Poliac, L.C. et al. *Sudden death in young competitive athletes: Clinical, demographic and pathological profiles.* JAMA 1996, 276: 199-204.
3. Van Camp, S.P., Bloor, C.M., Mueller, F.O. et al. *Nontraumatic sports death in high school and college athletes.* Med Sci Sports Exer 1995, 27: 641-7.
4. Burke, A.P., Farb, A., Virmani, R. et al. *Sports-related and non-sports-related sudden cardiac death in young athletes.* Am Heart J 1991, 121: 568-75.
5. Corrado, D., Thiene, G., Nava, A. et al. *Sudden death in young competitive athletes: Clinicopathologic correlations in 22 cases.* Am J Med 1990, 39: 588-96.
6. Maron, B.J., Roberts, W.C., McAllister, H.A. et al. *Sudden death in young athletes.* Circulation 1980, 62: 218-29.
7. Driscoll, D.J., Edwards, W.D. *Sudden unexpected death in children and adolescents.* J Am Coll Cardiol 1985, 5: 118B-21B.
8. Drory, Y., Turetz, Y., Hiss, Y. et al. *Sudden unexpected death in persons less than 40 years of age.* Am J Cardiol 1991, 68: 1388-92.
9. Liberthson, R.R. *Sudden death from cardiac causes in children and young adults.* N Engl J Med 1996, 334: 1039-44.
10. Maron, B.J., Epstein, S.E., Roberts, W.C. *Causes of sudden death in the competitive athlete.* J Am Coll Cardiol 1986, 7: 204-14.
11. Virmani, R., Robinowitz, M., McAllister, H.A. *Nontraumatic death in joggers. A series of 30 patients at autopsy.* Am J Med 1982, 72: 874-82.
12. Maron, B.J., Poliac, L.V., Kaplan, J.A. et al. *Blunt impact to the chest leading to sudden death from cardiac arrest during sports activities.* N Engl J Med 1995, 33: 337-42.
13. Maron, B.J., Strasburger, J.F., Kugler, J.D. et al. *Survival following blunt chest impact induced cardiac arrest during sports activities in young athletes.* Am J Cardiol 1997, 79: 840-41.
14. Link, M.S., Wang, P.J., Pandian, NG et al. *An experimental model of sudden death due to low-energy chest-wall impact (commotio cordis).* N Engl J Med 1998, 338: 1805-11.
15. Estes, N.A.M. III. *Sudden death in young athletes (editorial).* N Engl J Med 1995, 333: 380-81.
16. Maron, B.J., Gohman, T.E., Aeppli, D. *Prevalence of sudden cardiac death during competitive sports activities in Minnesota high school athletes.* J Am Coll Cardiol 1998, 32: 1881-4.

17. Maron, B.J., Mitchell, J.H. *26th Bethesda Conference. Recommendations for determining eligibility for competition in athletes with cardiovascular abnormalities.* J Am Coll Cardiol 1994, 24: 845-99.
18. Siscovick, D.S., Weiss, N.S., Fletcher, R.H. et al. *The incidence of primary cardiac arrest during vigorous exercise.* N Engl J Med 1984, 311: 874-7.
19. Thompson, P.D., Funk, E.J., Carleton, R.A. et al. *Incidence of death during jogging in Rhode Island from 1975 through 1980.* JAMA 1982, 247: 2535-8.
20. Thompson, P.D., Stern, M.P., Williams, P. et al. *Death during jogging or running. A study of 18 cases.* JAMA 1979, 242: 1265-7.
21. Maron, B.J., Poliac, L.C., Roberts, W.O. *Risk for sudden cardiac death associated with marathon running.* J Am Coll Cardiol 1996, 28: 428-31.
22. Maron, B.J., Kogan, J., Proschan, M.A., Hecht, G.M., Roberts, W.C. *Circadian variability in the occcurrence of sudden cardiac death in patients with hypertrophic cardiomyopathy.* J Am Coll Cardiol 1994, 23: 1405-9.
23. Maron, B.J., Poliac, L.C., Mathenge, R. *Hypertrophic cardiomyopathy as an important cause of sudden cardiac death on the athletic field in African-American athletes.* J Am Coll Cardiol 1997, 29 (Suppl. A): 462A.
24. Maron, B.J. *Heart disease and other causes of sudden death in young athletes.* Curr Probl Cardiol 1998, 23: 477-532.
25. Maron, B.J., Link, M.S., Wang, P.J., Estes N.A.M. *Clinical profile of commotio cordis: An under-appreciated cause of sudden death in the young during sports and other activities.* J Cardiovasc Electrophysiol 1999, 10: 114-20.
26. Maron, B.J., Thompson, P.D., Puffer, J.C. et al. *Cardiovascular preparticipation screening of competitive athletes.* Circulation 1996, 94: 850-6.
27. Pelliccia, A., Maron, B.J. *Preparticipation cardiovascular evaluation of the competitive athlete: Perspectives from the 30 year Italian experience.* Am J Cardiol 1995, 75: 827-8.
28. Corrado, D., Basso, C., Schiavon, M., Thiene G. *Screening for hypertrophic cardiomyopathy in young athletes.* N Engl J Med 1998, 339: 364-9.

CHAPTER 2

THE ITALIAN CLASSIFICATION OF DIFFERENT SPORTS IN RELATION TO CARDIOVASCULAR RISK

A. Dal Monte
Institute of Sports Science of the Italian National Olympic Committee

Cardiovascular risk in sports activities is highly correlated with the genetic characteristics of the athlete and the specific effort required to perform different kinds of sports. Sports activities evidently require a highly differentiated level of workload and length of energy expenditure. To define the cardiovascular impact produced by different sports and sports disciplines, we have to take into account the fact that the influence of sport activity on the heart depends more on training activity than on games or competitive events.

Different reasons for classifying sports activities in relation to cardiovascular function include: i) to define what kind of stress is produced by the different muscular exercises and the varied pattern of movements and repetition of movements on the human organism; ii) to verify what kind of adaptations and adjustments sport produces on the mechanics, morphology and biochemistry of the human body; and iii) to determine the way the heart and circulatory system react to sports requirements in acute and chronic adjustments.

Formulas such as "lightly trained", "average trained" or "highly trained", which are frequently adopted in the medical literature to differentiate sedentary people from the active population and from athletes, are clearly very unsatisfactory for defining cardiovascular risk.

Differences in training sessions and the involvement of the locomotion system are so varied, not only in physiology, biomechanics and biochemistry but also in cardiology, that it is necessary to refer to a more detailed classification in order to determine more precisely how the types of cardiovascular work weigh on the athlete.

In order to develop a practical classification of the influence of different sports on cardiovascular risk, it is useful to start from a physiological and biomechanical classification of sports, which takes into account six different groups of sports activities.

In the physiological-biomechanical classification (1), the different sports are divided into six categories. The criteria for this division are the physiological and biomechanical characteristics necessary for the athlete to achieve maximum results during competitive events. This classification has three fundamental criteria: the activated energy sources, the percentage of the total muscle mass used and the percentage of strength required by the involved muscles in the actual movement.

A. Bayés de Luna et al. (eds.), Arrhythmias and Sudden Death in Athletes, 11–24.
© 2000 *Kluwer Academic Publishers. Printed in the Netherlands.*

In the biomechanical classification (2), the six different types of sports activity are: i) activities requiring mainly anaerobic effort lasting from 20 to 40-45 sec; ii) activities requiring a massive aerobic-anaerobic effort lasting from 40-45 sec to 4-5 min; iii) activities requiring mainly aerobic effort lasting more than 4-5 min; iv) activities requiring alternated anaerobic-aerobic effort, the characteristic being the alternating phases of very intense effort (which is defined in terms of its anaerobic energy source whether it be the alactacid or nonacid lactic type); v) activities requiring great power, namely sports of a very brief duration, entirely involving the nonacid lactic anaerobic energy sources (the system: $ATP \rightarrow ADP + P$ and $ADP + CP \rightarrow ATP + C$), such as those with a strength effort (weight lifting), those with an impulse effort (throwing), and those with a propulsive effort (jumping and sprinting); and vi) activities requiring great skill, which are subdivided into activities requiring considerable muscular effort and a proper corporeal position (the effort required to control a vehicle or animal and also that needed to maintain a correct position) and activities requiring very little but very precise muscular movement (target shooting).

This classification is a sufficiently complete representation of the different sports activities. However, it gives no indication of heart participation and in particular no consideration for the heart rate cost. It is important to remember that this parameter is the easiest to obtain both on the field and in the laboratory.

On the basis of these six categories, a classification was formulated in 1969 and subsequently enriched by Lubich in 1990 (3), with the introduction of more modern sports, including some sports activities that were practiced infrequently (Tables 1-10). This classification takes into account the effort required in competitive events but not those required of the human body during training. The acute adjustments and chronic adaptations made by the heart and cardiovascular system do not depend on the effort made during competitions, which represents a very low percentage of the total time that athletes dedicate to sports activity. It is the training that is carried out for at least several hours a day, eleven months a year, year after year that requires cycles of very different workloads.

Table 1. General classification of sports activities. Adapted from (3).

Activities with chiefly anaerobic alactacid demands (strength sports)
Activities with chiefly anaerobic lactic acid demands
Activities with massive anaerobic aerobic demands
Activities with alternate aerobic anaerobic demands
Activities with chiefly aerobic demands
Activities requiring dexterity:
                         a) with considerable muscular demands
                         b) with few muscular demands
                         c) with postural and directional muscular demands
Activities with combined demands

Table 2. Activities with chiefly anaerobic nonacid lactic demands (strength sports). Adapted from (3).

Sports with chiefly strength demands:	Weight lifting (1, 4)
Sports with chiefly impelling demands:	Field athletics:
	Discus (1, 4)
	Hammer (1, 4)
	Javelin (1, 4)
	Shot put (1 ,4)

Sports with chiefly propulsive demands:	A. Antigravity	B. Orthogonal to gravity pull
	Track and field athletics	Track and field athletics
	High jump (1, 4)	100 m sprint (1, 4)
	Pole vault (1, 4)	110 m hurdles (1, 4)
	Long jump (1, 4)	
	Triple jump (1, 4)	
		Cycling
		Individual sprint (1, 4)
		Tandem sprint (1, 4)

Percentage muscular mass engaged: 1) +++ 2) ++ 3) +
District muscular strength required: 4) +++ 5) ++ 6) +

Table 3. Activities with chiefly anaerobic acid lactic demands (duration: 20-45 sec). Adapted from (3).

Track and field athletics:	200 m (1, 4)
	400 m (1, 4)
Body building (1, 4)	
Ice skating:	500 m sprint (1, 4)
Roller skating:	300 m timed (1, 4)
Cycling:	BMX track (1, 4)
Swimming:	50 m (1, 4)
Fin swimming:	50 m apnea (1, 4)
	100 m sub (1, 4)

Percentage muscular mass engaged: 1) +++ 2) ++ 3) +
District muscular strength required: 4) +++ 5) ++ 6) +

Table 4. Activities with massive anaerobic aerobic demands (duration: 45 sec to 5 min). Adapted from (3).

Swimming:	100 m (1, 4)	Track and field athletics:	800 m (1, 4)
	200 m (1, 4)		1,500 m (1, 4)
	400 m (1, 4)		400 m hurdles (1, 4)
Fin swimming:	200 m sup (1, 4)	Arm wrestling (2, 4)	
	400 m sup (1, 4)	Ice skating:	1,000 m (1, 4)
	400 m sub (1, 4)		1,500 m (1, 4)
Rowing (1,000 m women):	Individual (1, 4)		3,000 m (2, 4)
	Two pair (1, 4)	Roller skating:	500 m pursuit (1, 4)
	Two coxless (1, 4)		1,500 m (1, 4)
	Four with cox (1, 4)	Cycling:	Individual pursuit (1, 4)
	Four pair (1, 4)		Team pursuit (1, 4)
	Eight (1, 4)		Km from standing start (1, 4)
Canoeing (500 m	Kayak K1-K2-K4 (2, 4)		Keirin (1, 4)
and 1,000 m):	Canadian C1-C2 (2, 4)	Tug-o-war (1, 4)	

Percentage muscular mass engaged: 1) +++ 2) ++ 3) +
District muscular strength required: 4) +++ 5) ++ 6) +

Table 5. Activities with alternate aerobic anaerobic demands. Adapted from (3).

Soccer (1, 4)	Water polo (1, 5)
Five-a-side (1, 4)	*Tamburello* (1, 4)
Tennis (1, 4)	Boxing (1, 4)
Badminton (1, 5)	French boxing (1, 4)
Squash (1, 5)	Cycling: 100 km timed teams (2, 4)
Lacrosse (1, 5)	individual track points (2, 4)
Korfball (1, 5)	Ice hockey (1, 5)
Baseball (1, 4)	Lawn hockey (1, 5)
Softball (1, 4)	Roller skate hockey (1, 5)
Cricket (1, 5)	Hurling (1, 5)
Volleyball (1, 5)	American football (1, 4)
Handball (1, 5)	Rugby (1, 4)
Canoe polo (2, 4)	Dogsledding (1, 4)
Basque pelota (1, 4)	Wrestling:Greco-Roman (1, 4)
Pallone a bracciale (1, 5)	Free (1, 4)
Palla elastica (1, 5)	Catch (1, 4)
Basketball (1, 4)	Sumo (1, 4)

Percentage muscular mass engaged: 1) +++ 2) ++ 3) +
District muscular strength required: 4) +++ 5) ++ 6) +

Table 6. Activities with chiefly aerobic demands (duration in excess of 5 min). Adapted from (3).

Nordic skiing:	15 km (1 ,5)	Track and field athletics:	3,000 m steeplechase (1, 4)
	30 km (1, 5)		5,000 m (1, 4)
	50 km (1, 5)		10,000 m (1, 5)
			20 and 50 km walk (1, 5)
Ski roll (1,5)			
			Marathon (2, 5)
Swimming:	800 m (1, 4)		
	1,500 m (1, 5)	Rowing (2000m):	Individual (1, 4)
	Marathon (1, 5)		Two pair (1, 4)
			Four pair (1, 4)
			Two with cox (1, 4)
Fin swimming:	800 m sub (1, 4)		Two coxless (1, 4)
	800 m sup (1, 4)		Four with cox (1, 4)
	1,500m sup (1, 5)		For coxless (1, 4)
			Eight (1, 4)
Cycling:	Road (2, 4)		
	Stayer (2, 4)	Alpine skiing (1, 4)	
	Cyclecross (1, 4)		
	Mountain bike-MTB (1, 4)	Mountaineering	Free climbing (1, 5)
Ice skating:	5,000 m (1, 5)	Roller skating:	3,000 m (1, 4)
	10,000 m (1, 5)		5,000 m (2, 5)
	Trekking (2, 5)		10,000 m (2, 5)
			20,000 m (2, 5)
Triathlon:	(classic) (1, 4)		
	182 km cycling	Canoeing (10,000 m)	Kayak K1-K2-K4 (2, 4)
	+42 km running		Canadian C1-C2 (2, 4)
	+ 4 km swimming		Marathon K1-K2–C2 (2,5)

Percentage muscular mass engaged: 1) +++ 2) ++ 3) +
District muscular strength required: 4) +++ 5) ++ 6) +

Table 7. Activities requiring dexterity and making considerable muscular demands. Adapted from (3).

Water skiing:	Figure (1, 5)	Cycling:	Cycle-ball (1, 5)
	Slalom (1, 5)		Trialsin (1, 4)
	Jumps (1, 5)		Artistic cycling (1, 5)
	Barefoot jumps (1, 5)		BMX-freestyle (1, 5)
	Speed (1, 5)	Diving:	3 m board (1, 4)
Grass skiing (1, 5)			10 m board (1, 4)
Sand skiing (1, 5)		Canoeing:	Slalom (2, 5)
Alpine skiing:	Free (1, 4)		Rapids (2, 5)
	Slalom (1, 4)	Ice skating:	Artistic (1, 5)
	Combination (1, 4)		Rhythmic (1, 5)
	Km moving start (1, 5)	Martial arts	
Acrobatic skiing (1, 4)		without arms:	Judo (1, 5)
Extreme skiing (1, 4)			Jujitsu (1, 5)
Fencing:	Sword (1, 5)		Karate (1, 5)
	Foil (1, 5)		Tae kwon do (1, 4)
	Sabre (1, 5)		Kung fu (1, 5)
Synchronized			Aikido (1, 5)
swimming (1, 5)		Martial arts with arms:	Kendo (1, 5)
Polo (1, 5)			Kubudo (1, 5)
Orienteering (2,5)			Nunchaku (1, 5)
Windsurfing (1, 4)			Sai (1, 5)
Rafting (2, 4)		Gymnastics:	Artistic (1, 4)
Speleology (1, 5)			Apparatus (1, 4)
Mountaineering:	Rock climbing (1, 4)	Sports dancing (1, 5)	
	Ice climbing (1, 4)	Twirling (1, 5)	
	Free climbing (1, 4)		

Percentage muscular mass engaged: 1) +++ 2) ++ 3) +
+District muscular strength required: 4) +++ 5) ++ 6) +

Table 8. Activities requiring dexterity and making few muscular demands. Adapted from (3).

Target-shooting:	Smallbore free rifle (3, 6)
	Smallbore free rifle 3 positions (3, 6)
	Air rifle (3, 6)
	Free pistol (3, 5)
	Automatic pistol (3, 5)
	Bobbing target (3, 6)
	Practical shooting (2, 5)
Crossbow shooting:	Ancient (3, 5)
	Modern (3, 5)
Line fishing (3, 6)	
Croquet (3, 6)	
Clay-pigeon shooting:	Trapshooting (3, 6)
	Skeet (3, 6)
Frisbee (2, 5)	
Bowls (3, 6)	
Hunting (2, 5)	

Percentage muscular mass engaged: 1) +++ 2) ++ 3) +
District muscular strength required: 4) +++ 5) ++ 6) +

Table 9. Activities requiring dexterity and making postural and directional muscular demands. Adapted from (3).

Archery (2, 4)	Rally (3, 5)	Formula 1-2-3 (3, 6)
Table tennis (1, 5)	Endurance (3, 6)	Inboard-outboard (3, 6)
Surfing (1, 5)	Autocross (2, 4)	Offshore (3, 6)
Bowling (2, 5)	Jeeps (3, 5)	Hovercraft (3, 6)
Curling (2, 5)	Dragster (3, 6)	Yachting (Olympic):
Golf (3, 5)	Karting (3, 5)	Soling (2, 5)
Rodeoing (1, 4)	Vintage cars (2, 6)	Star (2, 5)
Parachuting (3, 6)	Bobcar (3, 5)	Tornado (2, 5)
Paraskiing (2, 5)	Sports flying:	Flying Dutchman (2, 5)
Hanggliding (3, 6)	Gliding (3, 6)	470 (2, 5)
Skjoring (2, 5)	Free flying (3, 6)	Horse-riding:
Monoskiing (2, 5)	Motor plane (3, 6)	Dressage (1, 5)
Skibobbing (3, 6)	Ultralight motor (3, 6)	Combined (1, 5)
Snowboarding (2, 4)	Hot-air balloon (3, 6)	Show jumping (1, 5)
Ski jumping (1, 5)	Windsurfing on snow (2, 5)	Noncompetitive
Motorcycling:	Sailing on ice (2, 5)	horseback-riding (2, 6)
Speed (3, 5)	Sailing on sand (2, 5)	Foxhunting (2, 5)
Motocross (1, 4)	Moto-waterskiing (1, 5)	Horse-and-carriage
Dirt bikes-ATV-Quad (1, 5)	Moto-sledding (2, 5)	racing (3, 6)
Trial (1, 4)	Hydrospeeding (2, 5)	Horse racing:
Enduro (2, 5)	Skateboarding (1, 5)	Trot (2, 6)
Endurance (2, 5)	Sledding:	Gallop (2, 6)
Speedway (1, 5)	Individual (2, 5)	Steeple-chasing (2, 5)
Motoball (1, 5)	Pair (2, 5)	Underwater activity:
Dragster (3, 6)	Skeleton (2, 5)	Skindiving (1, 5)
Moto-climbing (1, 5)	Bobsledding:	Photo safari (1, 5)
Motor racing:	Pair (2, 5)	Orienteering (1, 5)
Formula 1-2-3 (3, 5)	Foursome (2, 5)	
Formula free (3, 6)	Motorboat racing:	

Percentage muscular mass engaged: 1) +++ 2) ++ 3) +
District muscular strength required: 4) +++ 5) ++ 6) +

Table 10. Activities with combined demands. Adapted from (3).

Track and field athletics:	Decathlon: 100 m, long jump, shot put, 400 m, 100 m hurdles, discus, pole vault, javelin, 1,500 m, high jump (1, 4)
	Heptathlon: 100 m hurdles, shot put, high jump, 200 m, long jump, javelin, 800 m (1, 4)
Biathlon:	Nordic skiing, target-shooting (1, 5)
Modern pentathlon:	Show jumping, fencing, swimming, target-shooting, cross-country (1, 4)
Nordic combination:	Nordic skiing, ski jumping (1, 4)
Military pentathlon:	War course, cross-country, swimming, grenade throwing, rifle-shooting (1, 4)
Survival:	Land, sea, winter (1, 4)
War games:	Splash contact (1, 5)

Percentage muscular mass engaged: 1) +++ 2) ++ 3) +
District muscular strength required: 4) +++ 5) ++ 6) +

In order to classify cardiovascular risk in the different sports activities, it is of fundamental importance to know what kind of exercise athletes practice in their training sessions. For example, on the track and in the field the performance of the 100-meter sprinter lasts about 10 seconds or less, which means that peak heart frequency is reached after the end of the competition and that the cardiovascular impact is quite low. The training of a sprinter, on the other hand, requires very hard isotonic, isometric and eccentric maximal exercises, together with the use of very sophisticated gymnastic equipment. This kind of exercise produces a very high increase in blood pressure and sometimes very high peaks in heart frequency. In sprinting, as in several other competitive activities, the cardiocirculatory workload during the different macrocycles and microcycles that take place during preparation is much higher than in the competition itself.

Turning to long distance events, during competition the cardiocirculatory workload is high but submaximal and at a constant level of intensity. The situation is very different during training where, to improve the average speed and resistance at high speed, athletes carry out exercises based on several repetitions of very intense and lengthy prolonged efforts and consequently the cardiovascular workload is very high.

Sometimes the effect of sports on cardiovascular function is reflected in a very high heart frequency that is produced not by very intense energy expenditure but by emotional factors.

We consider that it is important for cardiologists to have especially detailed information about the specific impact on the cardiovascular system produced by different sports activities. However, at the same time, we must remember that such information is not designed for practical application in the clinical evaluation during routine cardiological controls.

The importance of classifying sports on the basis of workload, endurance and kind of movement has been taken into account by several authors when defining the amount of stress on the heart and vascular system. For the purposes of comparison, the classification of sports activities proposed by Mitchell *et al.* (4), which differs from that described above, may be used. In this classification, exercise is divided into dynamic and static (Table 11). Dynamic exercise involves changes in muscle length and joint movement with rhythmic contractions that develop a relatively small intramuscular force; static exercise involves the development of a relatively large intramuscular force with little or no change in muscle length or joint movement.

Both from a physiological and from a biomechanical point of view, the proposed basis of sports classification seems to be really pragmatic. It is particularly the definition of static that, probably because of the meaning that this term acquires in Italian, does not seem appropriate to define the kind of movement that it refers to. In my opinion, the only sports activity that can be considered static is target shooting. According to Mitchell *et al.*'s classification, weight lifting is static: it is hard for me to accept that weight lifting, which is based on very fast and ample angular movements of the principal joints and which requires maximal strength in a large number of muscles can be considered as static. Naturally, Mitchell's classification deserves maximum consideration but the definitions "low dynamic", "moderate dynamic", "high dynamic", "low static", "moderate static" and "high static" do not seem to accurately reflect what really happens in athletes trained in different sports disciplines.

Table 11. Sports classification (based on peak dynamic and static components during competition). Adapted from (4).

	A. Low dynamic	B. Moderate dynamic	C. High dynamic
I. Low static	Billiards Bowling	Baseball Softball	Badminton Cross-country skiing (classic technique)
	Cricket Curling Golf Riflery	Table tennis Tennis (doubles) Volleyball	Field hockey* Orienteering Race walking Racquetball Running (long distance) Soccer* Squash Tennis (single)
II. Moderate static	Archery Auto racing*§ Diving*§	Fencing Field events (jumping) Figure skating*	Basketball* Ice hockey* Cross-country skiing (skating technique)
	Equestrian*§ Motorcycling*§	Football (American)* Rodeoing*§ Rugby* Running (sprint) Surfing*§ Synchronized swimming§	Football (Australian rules)* Lacrosse* Running (middle distance) Swimming Team handball
III. High static	Bobsledding*§ Field events (throwing) Gymnastics*§ Karate/judo* Luge*§ Sailing Rock climbing*§ Waterskiing*§ Weight lifting*§ Windsurfing*§	Body building*§ Downhill skiing*§ Wrestling*	Boxing* Canoeing/kayaking Cycling*§ Decathlon Rowing Speed skating

* Danger of body collision.   § Increased risk if syncope occurs.

On the other hand, the same authors describe their classification based on peak dynamic and static components during competition. We do not consider that the cardiovascular risk is correlated with the acute adjustments that occur during competition; rather, they are correlated with the more intense and very prolonged and repeated stress that the athletes undergo during the different phases of training.

Competition stress can stimulate the human body to try to surpass the performance achieved during training. However, it is not taking part in competitions that produces the acute adjustments and chronic adaptations that characterize not only the variable geometry apparatus, which is the locomotion apparatus of the athlete, but also the cardiocirculatory system. It training, in particular, which is mostly based on several repetitions of very intense and highly stressful exercises, that produces the maximal variations in the cardiocirculatory system and consequently produces the cardiovascular risk.

Mitchell *et al.*(4) are very honest in evaluating their classification and in declaring its limitations. Their discussion of the different emotional and hormonal effects that may occur during competitions can be totally agreed with.

In an attempt to prepare a classification that takes into account the relationship between sport activities and cardiovascular demands, the Cardiological Organizing Committee for suitability for participation in competitive sports (COCIS) formulated some especially useful protocols for cardiologists to use when assessing athletes' suitability to participate in competitive sports (5, 6).

In the classification of Mitchell *et al.* (4) (Table 12), sports are classified also according to cardiocirculatory effort based on the dynamic muscular demands and, finally, on high neurosensorial demands. This classification can also be criticized on the basis of its definition of static and dynamic, which does not seem to correctly represent the work performed by the cardiovascular system. This is primarily expressed during training sessions and only secondarily during competition.

Notwithstanding the considerable difficulties inherent in classifying cardiovascular risk, it is important to try to study a simple classification, less sophisticated than those normally used by physiologists and biomechanics, one specifically created for cardiologists, in order to identify the cardiovascular system's workload.

As an alternative to the classification of Mitchell *et al.* (4) ours is based on the following parameters: heart frequency, cardiac output and mean arterial blood pressure. Thus, the classification directly takes into account the level of risk on the heart and circulatory system created by training and competitive events. This sports activities classification is subdivided into five groups, identifying: i) noncompetitive sports activities making minimum to moderate cardiocirculatory demands characterized by constant pumping activity, submaximal heart rate and the decline of peripheral resistance (Table 13); ii) sports activities making "neurogenous" cardiocirculatory demands characterized by increases in heart rate but not of output, owing to an important emotional impact, especially in competitions (Table 14); iii) sports activity making "pressure" cardiocirculatory demands, characterized by nonmaximal cardiac output, high or maximum heart rate and medium to high peripheral resistance (Table 15); iv) sport activities making medium to high cardiocirculatory demands, characterized by numerous and rapid (possibly maximum) increases in heart rate and output, with an increase in peripheral resistance particularly evident in the sudden interruption of the muscular activity of the limbs (Table 16) and; v) sports activities making high cardiocirculatory demands, characterized by pumping activity with maximum heart rate and maximum central and peripheral cardiac output (conditioned in duration by metabolic adaptation) (Table 17).

Clearly, we cannot use the definition of professional and amateur athletes to indicate cardiovascular risk. Currently, some amateur athletes receive no financial compensation and are therefore unconnected to any professional activity. Nevertheless, they follow training programs characterized by extremely hard and prolonged exercises. This kind of exercise is of the same intensity, if not harder, as the training sessions undertaken by some professional athletes.

Table 12. Classification of sporting activities in relation to cardiovascular demands according to COCIS – Cardiological protocols for assessing suitability of participating in competitive sports. Adapted from (5).

	A. With chiefly dynamic muscular demands	B. With chiefly static or explosive muscular demands	C. Making high neurosensorial demands
I. Sports with medium or high cardiovascular demands	Nordic skiing (cross-country skiing, biathlon, Nordic combined) Track cycling (pursuit and middle distance) and on road, cyclo-cross Running (extended sprints, middle distance, long distance, very long distance, cross-country) Rowing, canoeing (all specialties) Swimming, water polo Track or ice skating (long distance) Modern pentathlon Triathlon (swimming, cycling, long-distance running) Decathlon Squash Soccer, rugby, basketball, handball Hockey (on grass, ice and using roller skates) Tennis Beach-volley Skin-diving	American football Wrestling, boxing, full-contact, martial arts, fencing Track cycling (sprint) Sprint hurdling Weightlifting, field athletics (throwing, jumping) Artistic gymnastics, diving Alpine skiing (downhill, giant, slalom), sled, bob, mountaineering Water skiing, wind-surfing Motocross	
II. Sports with moderate cardiovascular demands	Table tennis, badminton, "tamburello" Volleyball Artistic skating	Baseball, softball	Piloting (of cars, motorcycles, aircraft, hang-gliders, para-chuting, motor-boats)
III. Sports with minimum cardiovascular demands	Golf, cricket, bowls, bowling Shooting sports (target-shooting, clay-pigeon shooting) Angling	Sailing Equestrian sports, horse racing, polo Archery	

Table 13. Noncompetitive sports activities with minimum to moderate cardiocirculatory demands characterized by constant pumping activity, submaximal heart rate and decline of peripheral resistance. Adapted from (6).

Running or walking on flat ground	Nordic skiing
Roadwork	Skating
Jogging	Noncompetitive canoeing
Cycling on flat ground	Trekking (not excessive)
Swimming	Golf
Hunting	

Table 14. Sports activities having "neurogenous" cardiocirculatory demands characterized by increases in heart rate (HR) but not in output, owing to an important emotional impact, especially in competitive events. Adapted from (6).

A. With medium-high HR increases	B. With minimum-moderate HR increases
Diving	Parachuting
Speed motorcycling	Golf
Motor racing	Bowls and bowling
Sports flying	Angling
Motorboat racing	Shooting sports (target, clay pigeon, archery, etc.)
Sailing	
Equestrian sports and polo	
Horse racing	
Underwater activities	

Table 15. Sport activities with pressure cardiocirculatory demands, characterized by nonmaximal cardiac output, high or maximum heart rate and medium-high peripheral resistance. Adapted from (6).

Track athletics (sprinting)	Heptathlon: throwing and jumping
Bobsledding	Skiing: slalom and downhill,
Sledding	km moving start
Cycling sprint and keirin	acrobatic skiing
Swimming 50 m	Waterskiing
Fin swimming: 50 m apnea, 100 m sub	Windsurfing
Ice skating (sprinting)	Table tennis
Roller skating (sprinting)	Motorcycling, motocross
Weightlifting	Mountaineering
Throwing	Free climbing
Jumping	Synchronized swimming
Decathlon: throwing and jumping	Body building

Table 16. Sports activities with medium to high cardiocirculatory demands, characterized by numerous and rapid (possibly maximum) increases in heart rate and output, with an increase in peripheral resistance particularly evident in the sudden interruption of the muscular activity of limbs. Adapted from (6).

Soccer	Water polo	Tennis	Boxing
Five-a-side soccer	Baseball	Canoeing slalom	Ice hockey
American football	Softball	Squash	Court hockey
Rugby	Cricket	Badminton	Lawn hockey
Basketball	Beach volleyball	*Tamburello*	Artistic skating
Volleyball	Artistic gymnastics	Martial arts	
Handball	Fencing	Wrestling	

Table 17. Sports activities with high cardiocirculatory demands, characterized by pumping activity with maximum heart rate and maximum central and peripheral cardiac output (conditioned in duration by the metabolic adaptation. Adapted from (6).

Field and track athletics:
  400 m, 400 m hurdles, 800 m, 1,500 m, 3,000 m steeplechase, 5,000 m, 10,000 m, marathon, 20 km and 50 km walk
Canoeing: 500 m, 1,000 m, 10,000 m, marathon – all craft
Rowing all craft
Cycling:
  individual and team pursuit, points race, km from starting point, line, individual time, mountain bike (cross country and downhill) and cyclecross
Decathlon: running only
Heptathlon: running only
Swimming: 100 m, 200 m, 400 m, 800 m, 1,500 m, marathon
Fin swimming: 400 m and 800 m sub, 200 m, 400 m, 800 m and 1,500 m sup
Ice skating: 500 m, 1,500 m, 30,000 m, 5,000 m, 10,000 m
Roller skating: 500 m, 1,500 m, 30,000 m, 5,000 m, 10,000 m, 20,000 m
Pentathlon: running and swimming
Alpine skiing: giant slalom, super G
Nordic skiing: 15 km, 30 km, 50 km
Biathlon (skiing, target-shooting)
Classic triathlon

The effect of training sessions on the human body, and particularly on the cardiovascular system, depends on different factors: in particular, the age at which athletes start training and the kind of performance for which they are prepared. Also, the length of an athlete's career does not always represent a negative effect; sometimes it represents a positive effect in terms of strengthening of the cardiovascular system. For example, swimmers start their sports activity very early, several years before the body is fully developed, which means that they start very heavy training sessions at about 9-10 years of age. After 10 years of training, when they reach the age of about 20 years, we could imagine finding very extensive modifications in the total heart dimensions and an increase in the cardiac walls. Twenty or thirty years ago, very enlarged hearts were found in athletes who had begun to train during or after puberty. Today, we can verify that, probably due to the complete adaptation of the central and peripheral circulation, which takes place when training starts at a very early age, the peripheral circulation and capillary growth are so intense that, during hard training sessions, blood pressure does not increase but peripheral resistance does. This indicates that the training process produces a very beneficial effect on the heart because the pump can send a large amount of blood to the peripheral regions, mainly the arms and legs, without the need to increase blood pressure. Consequently, there is improved vascularization in the heart's muscular system, *i.e.*, the wall muscles, but without an increase in its muscular mass thickness. Nowadays, echocardiography shows that in top level swimmers, after 15-20 years of hard training, the heart is not particularly overenlarged and that the heart walls are developed harmoniously, according to the increase in the left and the right ventricular chamber.

Generally, in sports like cycling, which require very severe and prolonged efforts, as well as in climbing training, which requires maximal cardiac output and a very high increase in peripheral blood pressure, we do not find a very big increase in the thickness of cardiac walls, which means that the workload does not bring about a high increase in the central blood pressure.

In rowers, very large bodied athletes, with very long training sessions (5 or 6 h/day), the relatively low frequency in the repetition of movements, 25-35 strokes/min, with the contemporaneous maximal contractions of the lower limbs extended and upper limbs contracted, gives an immediate increase in the peripheral blood pressure, which, of course, imposes a very high workload on the heart, both due to the need for maximal stroke volume and, at the same time, to very high blood pressure.

It must be taken into consideration that athletes often produce a spontaneous Valsalva during muscular gesture. In these athletes the heart's workload is maximal both in cardiac output and in blood pressure.

Rowers perform better than in the past but in this case the heart volumes are, of course, bigger than those of sedentary people, although they are not as big as those that we have in our x-ray archives, which contain the radiograms of athletes from 30-40 years ago. In addition, the early use of rigorous and prolonged training sessions produces global peripheral capillary growth and vascularization, which reduces the heart's workload and, consequently, the heart's muscle size is not overly increased.

It should also be taken into account that although rowers' movements can be compared to those of weight lifters performing not only in a vertical but also in a horizontal position, rowers also train by undertaking other kinds of exercises (such as running, climbing, jumping) and by using very sophisticated equipment in the gym.

The situation is very different for weight lifters that base their training on a relatively small number of exercise repetitions that require a very high percentage of their maximal muscular strength. Younger weight lifters do not train in this way; maximal intensity exercises are undertaken at around the age of puberty. In this kind of athlete, using the parameters of heart frequency, cardiac output and mean arterial blood pressure in our classification, we have to take into consideration that weight lifters produce very high mean arterial blood pressure but they do not produce high cardiac frequencies and cardiac output.

In conclusion, we consider that a classification specifically tailored to cardiologists should primarily consider the training efforts that are required during the different macrocycles and microcycles where a large variety of efforts are included. On this basis, we consider that the second COCIS classification, elaborated by representatives of multidisciplinary sport scientists (e.g. physiologists, biomechanics, cardiologists and training methodologists), even if it cannot be considered as a totally satisfactory, is the most balanced classification, capable of offering cardiologists more precise guidelines for the cardiological evaluation of athletes.

References

1. Dal Monte, A. *Proposta di una classificazione ad orientamento biomeccanico delle attività sportive.* Med Sport 1969, 22: 501-9.
2. Dal Monte A. *Physiological classification of sports activities and cardiovascular function* In: Sports Cardiology. A. Venerando, T. Lubich (Eds.). Aulo Gaggi Edit.: Bologna 1980: 161-99.

3. Lubich, T., Cesaretti, D. *Revisione, proposte di inquadramento e classificazione delle attività sportive.* Med Sport 1990, 43: 223-9.

4. Mitchell, J.H., Haskell, W., Raven P.B. *Classification of sports.* 26th Bethesda Conference Report. JACC 1994, 24: 864-6.

5. COCIS (Comitato Organizzativo Cardiologico per il giudizio di idoneità allo sport). *Protocolli cardiologici per il giudizio di idoneità allo sport agonistico.* Int J Sports Card 1988, 5: 62-87.

6. COCIS (Comitato Organizzativo Cardiologico per il giudizio di idoneità allo sport). *Protocolli cardiologici per il giudizio di idoneità allo sport agonistico 1995.* Int J Sports Card 1995, 4: 143-67.

CHAPTER 3

CLASSIFICATION OF SPORTS*

J.H. Mitchell, W.L. Haskell and P.B. Raven
*The University of Texas, Southwestern Medical Center at Dallas,
Department of Internal Medicine, Dallas, Texas, USA*

Competitive sports can place an athlete with a cardiovascular abnormality at medical risk because of an increase in work load on the heart or stress on the vascular system caused by increases in blood flow and pressure and increased body temperature. This may be reflected in an increased risk for sudden death, life-threatening cardiovascular alterations or disease progression.

Types of Exercise Performed

Sports can be classified according to the type and intensity of exercise performed and also with regard to the danger of bodily injury from collision or the consequences of syncope (1-3). Exercise can be divided into two broad types: dynamic and static (4,5). Dynamic exercise involves changes in muscle length and joint movement with rhythmic contractions that develop a relatively small intramuscular force; static exercise involves development of a relatively large intramuscular force with little or no change in muscle length or joint movement. These two types of exercise should be thought of as the two extremes of a continuum, with most physical activity having both static and dynamic components. For example, distance running has principally low static and high dynamic demands, whereas waterskiing has principally high static and low dynamic demands.

Dynamic exercise performed with a large muscle mass causes a marked increase in oxygen consumption (Fig. 1). There is a substantial increase in cardiac output, heart rate, stroke volume and systolic blood pressure; a moderate increase in mean arterial pressure; and a decrease in diastolic blood pressure. Also, there is a marked decrease in total peripheral resistance. Static exercise, on the other hand, causes a small increase in oxygen consumption, cardiac output and heart rate and no change in stroke volume (Fig. 1). Also, there is a marked increase in systolic, diastolic and mean arterial pressure and no appreciable change in total peripheral resistance. Thus, dynamic exercise primarily causes a volume load on the left ventricle, whereas static exercise causes a pressure load on the cardiovascular system. The cardiovascular responses during dynamic exercise of a small muscle mass at low resistance or during dynamic exercise of a large muscle mass at high resistance are similar to the responses during static exercise (6).

*Reprinted with permission from the American College of Cardiology (Journal of the American College of Cardiology, 1994, 24(4), 845-99).

A. Bayés de Luna et al. (eds.), Arrhythmias and Sudden Death in Athletes, 25–30.
© 2000 *Kluwer Academic Publishers. Printed in the Netherlands.*

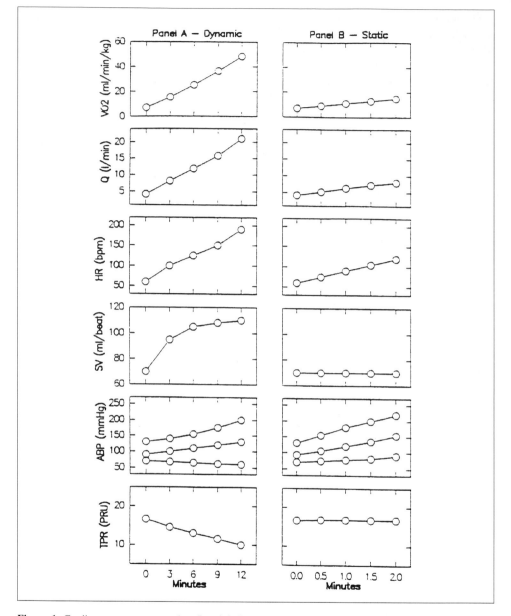

Figure 1. Cardiac response to exercise. *Panel A*, Response to dynamic exercise of progressively increasing work load to maximal oxygen consumption. *Panel B*, Response to a static handgrip contraction at 30% maximal voluntary contraction. ABP (mmHg) = systolic, mean and diastolic arterial blood pressures; HR (bpm) = heart rate (beats/min); Q (l/min) = cardiac output (liters/min); SV (ml/beat) = stroke volume; TPR (PRU) = total peripheral resistance in peripheral resistance units; VO2 (ml/min/kg) = oxygen consumption (ml/min x body weight in kg). From Mitchell JH. Raven PB. Cardiovascular adaptation to physical activity. In: Bouchard C, Shephard RJ, Stephens T, editors. Physical Activity, Fitness and Health: International Proceedings and Consensus Statement (Figure 17.2). Champaign (IL): Human Kinetics Publishers. Copyright 1994 by Human Kinetics Publishers, Inc. Reprinted with permission.

The terms *dynamic* and *static* exercise characterize activity on the basis of the mechanical action involved and are different from the terms *aerobic* and *anaerobic* exercise, which characterize activity on the basis of the type of metabolism. Most high intensity static exercise is performed primarily anaerobically, whereas high intensity dynamic exercise lasting for more than several minutes is performed primarily aerobically. However, dynamic exercise, such as sprinting or jumping, is performed primarily anaerobically. Thus, a wide variety of sports are placed in the high dynamic category, including such diverse activities as skiing (cross-country), running (distance), soccer and squash. Because the cardiovascular demands of very high resistance dynamic exercise are similar to sustained static exercise, those sports that have either a sustained static component or a very high resistance dynamic component are classified together as high intensity static exercise (weight lifting, gymnastics and field events [throwing]).

Cardiac Hypertrophy

Athletes who participate in sports with a high dynamic component have a larger absolute left ventricular mass and chamber size (eccentric hypertrophy) than sedentary subjects (7, 8). This eccentric hypertrophy develops gradually and correlates with maximal oxygen uptake (8). Athletes who participate in sports with a high static component also have a larger left ventricular mass but no increase in chamber size (concentric hypertrophy) (7, 8). This concentric hypertrophy is not associated with a high maximal oxygen uptake. Athletes who participate in sports with both high dynamic and high static demands (*e.g.*, rowing and cycling) have a combination of eccentric and concentric hypertrophy.

Myocardial Oxygen Demand

Both dynamic and static exercise change several factors that are important in determining myocardial oxygen demand: heart rate, wall tension and contractile state of the ventricle (9, 10). Wall tension is affected by pressure development and ventricular volume. In high intensity dynamic exercise, there is a large increase in heart rate and an increase in stroke volume that is achieved by both an increase in end-diastolic volume (Frank-Starling mechanism) and a decrease in end-systolic volume (increased contractile state). In high intensity static exercise there is a smaller increase in heart rate and little change in end-diastolic and end-systolic volumes of the left ventricle. However, arterial pressure and contractile state of the ventricle are increased. Thus, both dynamic and static exercise cause increases in factors that are important in determining myocardial oxygen demand.

Classification of Sports

A classification of sports is provided in Table 1, which classifies individual sports according to the two general types of exercise: dynamic and static (4-6). Each sport is classified by the level of intensity (low, medium, high) of dynamic and static exercise generally

Table 1. Classification of sports (based on peak dynamic and static components during competition)

	A. Low dynamic	B. Moderate dynamic	C. High dynamic
I. Low static	Billiards Bowling Cricket Curling Golf Riflery	Baseball Softball Table tennis Tennis (doubles) Volleyball	Badminton Cross-country skiing (classic technique) Field hockey* Orienteering Race walking Racquetball Running (long distance) Soccer* Squash Tennis (singles)
II. Moderate static	Archery Auto racing*† Diving*† Equestrian*† Motorcycling*†	Fencing Field events (jumping) Figure skating* Fontball (American)* Rodeoing*† Rugby* Running (sprint) Surfing*† Synchronized swimming†	Basketball* Ice hockey* Cross-country skiing (skating technique) Football (Australian rules)* Lacrosse* Running (middle distance) Swimming Team handball
III. High static	Bobsledding*† Field events (throwing) Gymnastics*† Karate/judo* Luge*† Sailing Rock climbing*† Waterskiing*† Weight lifting*† Windsurfing*†	Body building*† Downhill skiing*† Wrestling*	Boxing* Canoeing/kayaking Cycling* Decathlon Rowing Speed skating

*Danger of bodily collision. †Increased risk if syncope occurs.

required to perform that sport during competition. It also indicates those sports that pose significant danger due to bodily collision, either because of the probability of hard impact between competitors or between a competitor and an object and the degree of risk posed to the athlete or others if sudden syncope occurred. Thus, in terms of their dynamic and static demands, sports can be classified (see Table 1) as IIIC (high static, high dynamic), IIB (moderate static, moderate dynamic), IA (low static, low dynamic), and so forth. For example, an athlete with a cardiovascular disorder that contraindicates a sport that produces a high pressure load on the left ventricle may be advised to avoid sports classified as IIIA, IIIB and IIIC. It should be emphasized that in terms of the classification of sports matrix presented in Table 1, cardiovascular abnormalities designated as compatible with a high level of intensity in any particular category also (by definition) permit levels of lesser intensity. For example, if class IC is appropriate (low static/*high* dynamic), then so are classes IA and IB (low static/*low* and *moderate* dynamic).

Limitations of Classification

There are important limitations to the classification of sports according to the type and intensity of exercise performed, as presented in Table 1. For example, it does not consider the emotional stress that an athlete experiences during a competitive event, the effects of environmental factors or the specific training regimen used by the athlete. Also, for team sports the classification is based on the highest cardiovascular demands that are experienced during competition and does not consider the cardiovascular demands of a specific position. For example, there are large differences in the cardiovascular demands required during soccer competition for a midfielder compared with a goalkeeper.

During all athletic competition the emotional involvement of the athlete can substantially increase sympathetic drive, and the resulting catecholamine concentrations can increase blood pressure, heart rate and myocardial contractility, thereby increasing myocardial oxygen demand. Also, the increase in sympathetic tone can cause arrthymias and may aggravate existing myocardial ischemia. Thus, even in sports such as golf or riflery, which have low myocardial oxygen demands due to the exercise required, substantial increases may occur because of emotional involvement during competition. This problem needs to be considered in determining the eligibility for sports participation of athletes with existing cardiovascular abnormalities.

Environmental exposure during athletic competition or training needs to be considered. Performance at high altitudes or under water may decrease oxygen availability, whereas hot or cold temperatures and high humidity can increase myocardial work load for the same intensity of exercise. Another environmental factor that needs to be considered is air pollution, especially elevated carbon monoxide levels, in a sport such as auto racing.

With the modern application of exercise science to competitive sports, training for competition can be more demanding on the cardiovascular system than the competition itself. For some sports the training program requires a different type and increased intensity of exercise and thereby stress to the cardiovascular system. Many training regimens now use heavy resistance weight training (heavy resistance dynamic or static exercise) for increasing strength and power in sports that do not include heavy resistance or static exercise during competition (*e.g.*, tennis, basketball). In some cases, where it is found acceptable for the athlete to participate in the competitive aspect of a specific sport but the existing training program is considered too vigorous, it may be possible to modify the training so as to reduce the cardiovascular stress to an acceptable level.

Conclusions

Because our knowledge of the relative risks of the cardiovascular demands of static and dynamic exercise for athletes with various cardiovascular abnormalities is incomplete, this classification of sports must be regarded as largely theoretic. Nevertheless, it represents a reasonable estimate of the relative risks involved with various competitive sports and should have practical value.

References

1. Mitchell, J.H., Blomqvist, C.G., Haskell, W.L., et al. *Classification of sports. 16th Bethesda Conference. Cardiovascular abnormalities in the athlete: Recommendations regarding eligibility for competition.* J Am Coll Cardiol 1985, 6: 1198-9.
2. Shaffer, T.E. *The health examination for participation in sports.* Pediatr Ann 1978, 7: 666-75.
3. Strong, W.B., Alpert, B.S. *The child with heart disease: Play, recreation, and sports.* Curr Probl Cardiol 1981, 6: 1-38.
4. Mitchell, J.H., Wildenthal, K. *Static (isometric) exercise and the heart: Physiological and clinical considerations.* Ann Rev Med 1974, 25: 369-81.
5. Asmussen, E. *Similarities and dissimilarities between static and dynamic exercise.* Circ Res 1981, 48 (Suppl. 1): I-3-10.
6. Blomqvist, C.G., Lewis, S.F., Taylor, W.F., Graham, R.M. *Similarity of the hemodynamic responses to static and dynamic exercise of small muscle groups.* Circ Res 1981, 48 (Suppl. 1): I-87-92.
7. Pelliccia, A., Maron, B.J., Spataro, A., Proschan, M.A., Spirito, P. *The upper limit of physiologic cardiac hypertrophy in highly trained elite athletes.* N Engl J Med 1991, 324: 295-301.
8. Mitchell, J.H., Raven, P.B. *Cardiovascular adaptation to physical activity.* In: Physical Activity, Fitness and Health: International Proceedings and Consensus Statement. Bouchard, C., Shephard, R., Stephens, T. Human Kinetics: Champaign 1994: 286-98.
9. Sonnenblick, E.H., Ross, J. Jr., Braunwald, E. *Oxygen consumption of the heart: Newer concepts of its multifactorial determination.* Am J Cardiol 1968, 22: 328-36.
10. Mitchell, J.H., Hefner, L.L., Monroe, R.G. *Performance of the left ventricle.* Am J Med 1972, 53: 481-94.

CHAPTER 4

CARDIOVASCULAR CAUSES AND PATHOLOGY OF SUDDEN DEATH
IN ATHLETES: THE AMERICAN EXPERIENCE

B.J. Maron
Minneapolis Heart Institute Foundation, Minneapolis, Minnesota, USA

"The time you won your town the race
We chaired you through the market-place;
Man and boy stood cheering by,
And home we brought you shoulder high.

To-day, the road all runners come,
Shoulder-high we bring you home,
And set you at your threshold down,
Townsman of a stiller town."

-To An Athlete Dying Young
Alfred Edward Housmann, 1895

A large proportion of the population of the United States participates in athletic activi-ties, often involving systematic sports training and competition. Understandably, consid-erable interest has evolved regarding the sudden unexpected deaths of young (or older) athletes. These uncommon catastrophes, which often become highly visible events, usu-ally prove to be the consequence of a variety of unsuspected congenital or acquired car-diovascular diseases (1-15) and convey a devastating impact on the community (16).

The young, highly conditioned, competitive athlete projects the imagery of the health-iest facet of our society. Consequently, the recognition that athletic field deaths may be due to a variety of potentially detectable cardiovascular lesions has stimulated substan-tial interest in the criteria used to determine eligibility and disqualification from compet-itive sports (17, 18).

Causes of Sudden Death in Young Athletes

Several autopsy-based studies have described the cardiovascular diseases responsible for sudden death in young competitive athletes, or youthful asymptomatic individuals with active life-styles (1-15). These structural abnormalities are independent of the normal physiological adaptations in cardiac dimensions that appear to occur as a consequence of long-term, systematic training in many athletes.

31
A. Bayés de Luna et al. (eds.), Arrhythmias and Sudden Death in Athletes, 31–48.
ⓒ *2000 Kluwer Academic Publishers. Printed in the Netherlands.*

The vast majority of sudden deaths in young athletes (age ≤35) are due to a variety of primarily congenital cardiovascular diseases (over 20 in number) (Fig. 1, Table 1) (1-3, 8). Indeed, virtually any disease capable of causing sudden death in young people may potentially do so in young competitive athletes. It should be emphasized that each of these diseases are uncommon within the general population and many are even uncommon among young athletes dying suddenly, responsible for only ≤5% of all the tabulated deaths (Table 1) (1).

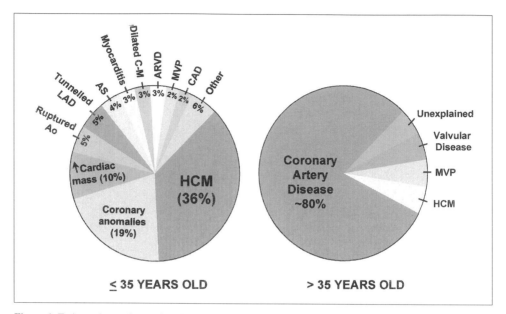

Figure 1. Estimated prevalence of cardiovascular diseases responsible for sudden death are compared in young (≤35 years old) and older (>35 years) trained athletes. *Left.* Causes of sudden cardiac death in young competitive athletes (median age, 17) based on systematic tracking of 158 athletes in the United States, primarily 1985-1995. In an additional 2% of the series, no evidence of cardiovascular disease sufficient to explain death was evident at autopsy. "Possible hypertrophic cardiomyopathy (HCM)" denotes those hearts with some morphological features consistent with (but not diagnostic of) HCM. Adapted from (1) with the permission of the American Medical Association. *Right.* Causes of sudden cardiac death in older trained athletes. Data shown here were assembled by collating findings from available published studies. ARVD = arrhythmogenic right ventricular dysplasia. AS = aortic stenosis. CAD = coronary artery disease. C-M = cardiomyopathy. LAD = left anterior descending coronary artery. LVH = left ventricular hypertrophy; MVP = mitral valve prolapse. Reproduced from (9) with the permission of the Journal of American College of Cardiology.

HYPERTROPHIC CARDIOMYOPATHY

The single most common cardiovascular disease responsible for sudden death in the young athlete is hypertrophic cardiomyopathy (HCM), usually in the nonobstructive form, and with a prevalence of about 35% (Figs. 1, 2, Table 1) (1, 2, 5, 8, 9). HCM is a primary and familial cardiac malformation with heterogeneous expression and a diverse clinical course for which several disease-causing mutations in nine genes encoding proteins of the sarcomere have been reported (19-26). HCM is a relatively common genetic disorder, occurring in 0.17% (about 1 in 500) of the general population (25).

Table 1. Cardiovascular abnormalities in 134 young competitive athletes with sudden death

Primary cardiovascular lesions	No.(%) of athletes	Median age (range), years
Hypertrophic cardiomyopathy (HCM)	48 (36.0)	17.0 (13-28)
Unexplained increase in cardiac mass§	14 (10.0)	17.0 (14-24)
(possible hypertrophic cardiomyopathy)		
Aberrant coronary arteries	17* (13.0)	15.0 (12-23)
Other coronary anomalies	8 (6.0)	17.5 (14-40)
Ruptured aortic aneurysm	6 (5.0)	17.0 (16-31)
Tunnelled LAD coronary artery	6 (5.0)	17.5 (14-20)
Aortic valve stenosis	6 (5.0)	14.0 (14-17)
Consistent with myocarditis	4 (3.0)	15.5 (13-16)
Idiopathic myocardial scarring	4 (3.0)	20.0 (14-27)
Idiopathic dilated cardiomyopathy	4 (3.0)	18.0 (18-21)
ARVD	4 (3.0)	16.0 (15-17)
Mitral valve prolapse	3 (2.0)	16.0 (15-23)
Atherosclerotic coronary artery disease	3 (2.0)	19.0 (14-28)
Other congenital heart diseases	2 (1.5)	13.5 (12-15)
Long QT syndrome	1 (0.5)	...
Sarcoidosis	1 (0.5)	...
Sickle cell trait[†]	1 (0.5)	...
"Normal" heart[‡]	3 (2.0)	18.0 (16-21)

LAD = left anterior descending. ARVD = arrhythmogenic right ventricular dysplasia. *Anomalous origin of left main coronary artery from right sinus of Valsalva in 13, anomalous origin of right coronary artery from left sinus of Valsalva in two, anomalous origin of the left main (from between the left and posterior cusps) with acute-angled take-off in one, and origin of left anterior descending coronary from pulmonary trunk in one.†Judged to be the probable cause of death in the absence of any identifiable structural cardiovascular abnormality.‡Absence of structural heart disease on standard autopsy examination.

In tertiary hospital and outpatient-based patient profiles, sudden death in HCM has shown a predilection for young and asymptomatic individuals and frequently during moderate or severe exertion, similar to its demographic profile as a frequent cause of death in athletic populations (27). Indeed, in a disease such as HCM in which there is a propensity for potentially lethal arrhythmias in some individuals, the stress of intense athletic training and competition (as well as associated alterations in blood volume, hydration and electrolytes) undoubtedly increases risk for a sudden event to some degree. On the other hand, some athletes with HCM appear to tolerate their disease over long periods of time, even when engaged in intense competitive sports (28).

Disease variables that appear to identify those HCM patients (or athletes) at the greatest risk include (21, 23): prior aborted cardiac arrest or sustained ventricular tachycardia; family history of sudden or other premature HCM-related deaths (and/or laboratory identification of a high-risk genotype); multiple-repetitive nonsustained ventricular tachycardia on ambulatory (Holter) ECG recording; recurrent syncope particularly if exertional and/or in the young; and massive degrees of left ventricular hypertrophy (Fig. 3). The magnitude of the left ventricular outflow gradient has also recently been associated with an increased risk for premature HCM-related heart failure death.

Left ventricular hypertrophy has traditionally been regarded as the gross anatomic marker and the likely determinant of many of the disease features and the clinical course

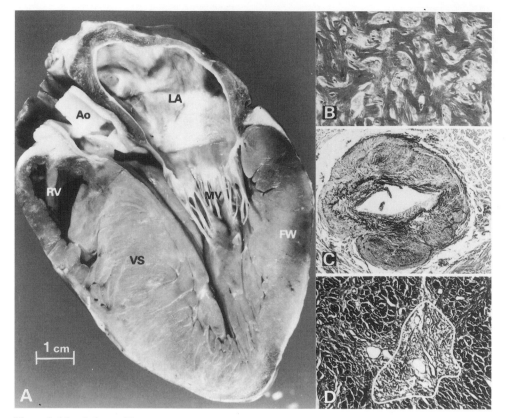

Figure 2. Morphology of hypertrophic cardiomyopathy (HCM), the most common cause of sudden death in young competitive athletes. Panel A shows a gross heart specimen sectioned in a cross-sectional plane similar to that of the echocardiographic (parasternal) long-axis; left ventricular wall thickening shows an asymmetric pattern and is confined primarily to the ventricular septum (VS) which bulges prominently into the left ventricular outflow tract. Left ventricular cavity appears reduced in size. FW = left ventricular free wall. B, C and D show histological features characteristic of left ventricular myocardium in HCM. B: markedly disordered architecture with adjacent hypertrophied cardiac muscle cells arranged at perpendicular and oblique angles. C: an intramural coronary artery with thickened wall (due primarily to medial hypertrophy) and apparently narrowed lumen. D: replacement fibrosis in an area of ventricular myocardium adjacent to an abnormal intramural coronary artery. Ao = aorta; LA = left atrium; RV = right ventricle. Reproduced with the permission of Lippincott-Raven Publishers from Maron, B.J. *Heart disease and other cardiovascular risks in competitive athletes*. In: Cardiology Parmley, W.W., Chatterje, K. (Eds.). 1997, 3: 1-19.

in most patients with HCM (Fig. 2) (19, 22-24). Since the left ventricular cavity is usually small or normal in size, increased left ventricular mass is due almost entirely to an increase in wall thickness. Consequently, the clinical diagnosis of HCM is based on the definition (by two-dimensional echocardiography) of the most characteristic morphological feature of the disease, *i.e.*, thickening of the left ventricular wall, usually asymmetrically, associated with a nondilated cavity, and in the absence of another cardiac or systemic disease capable of producing the magnitude of hypertrophy present, such as systemic hypertension or aortic stenosis) (29). Because the nonobstructive form of HCM is

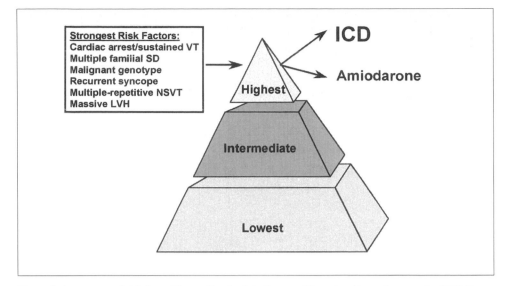

Figure 3. Assessment of risk for sudden cardiac death in the overall hypertrophic cardiomyopathy (HCM) population. Treatment for prevention of sudden death is limited to that small subset perceived to be at the highest risk compared to all other patients, with HCM, based on risk factor analysis. ICD = implantable cardioverter-defibrillator; LVH = left ventricular hypertrophy; NSVT = nonsustained ventricular tachycardia; SD = sudden death; VT = ventricular tachycardia.

predominant (19), the well-known clinical features of dynamic obstruction to left ventricular outflow, such as a loud systolic ejection murmur, systolic anterior motion of the mitral valve or partial premature closure of the aortic valve are not required for this diagnosis.

Based on both echocardiographic and necropsy analyses in large numbers of patients, it is apparent that the HCM disease spectrum is characterized by vast structural diversity with regard to the patterns and extent of left ventricular hypertrophy (22). Indeed, virtually all possible patterns of left ventricular hypertrophy occur in HCM, and no single phenotypic expression can be considered "classic" or typical of this disease (22, 30). While many patients show diffusely distributed hypertrophy, of note, fully 30% demonstrate localized and usually mild wall thickening confined to only one segment of the left ventricle. Absolute thickness of the left ventricular wall varies greatly, with the average reported value usually 21-22 mm (22). Wall thickness is profoundly increased in many patients, including some showing the most severe hypertrophy observed in any cardiac disease; 60 mm is the most extreme wall thickness dimension reported to date (31). On the other hand, the HCM phenotype is not invariably expressed as a greatly thickened left ventricle, and some patients show only a mild increase of ≤15 mm, including a very few genetically affected adult individuals with normal wall thickness (≤12 mm) (32, 33).

Hearts with increased mass (and wall thickness) and nondilated left ventricular cavity suggestive of HCM, but in which the objective morphological findings are not sufficiently striking to permit a definitive diagnosis of this disease, are not infrequently encountered at autopsy (Table 1) (1). It is uncertain whether these cases (sometimes

referred to as idiopathic left ventricular hypertrophy) (1, 5) represent a mild morphological expression of HCM, or possibly unusual instances of "athlete's heart" with particularly marked left ventricular hypertrophy and associated with deleterious consequences.

CONGENITAL CORONARY ARTERY MALFORMATIONS

Second in importance and frequency to HCM is a spectrum of congenital vascular malformations of the coronary arterial tree (occurring in about 20%), the most common of
which appears to be anomalous origin of the left main coronary artery from the right
(anterior) sinus of Valsalva with course between aorta and pulmonary trunk (Fig. 4) (1,
8, 34-41). Such coronary artery anomalies are difficult to identify because they may not
be readily identifiable by conventional noninvasive imaging technology, or simply
because they are exceedingly rare and the clinical index of suspicion is not always sufficiently high. Compounding this problem is the observation that the conventional resting
12-lead ECG and exercise ECG are usually within normal limits (without evidence of
myocardial ischemia) in the presence of an anomalous coronary artery from the wrong
aortic sinus (41).

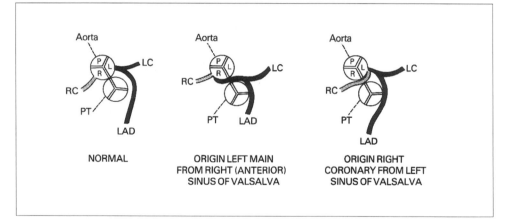

Figure 4. Congenital coronary artery anomalies capable of causing sudden death in young athletes. *Left.*
Normal anatomy is shown for comparison. *Center.* Anomalous origin of the left main coronary artery from the
right (anterior) sinus of Valsalva. The left coronary artery may have a separate or common ostium with the right
coronary artery, which also arises from the right (R) sinus of Valsalva. Note the acute leftward bend of the left
main coronary artery at its origin and its posterior course between the aorta and pulmonary trunk (PT). *Right.*
The right coronary (RC) artery arises anomalously from the left (L) coronary sinus in association with the left
main coronary artery and shows a similar acute bend at its origin before it courses between the great arteries.
LAD = left anterior descending coronary artery; LCV = left anterior descending coronary artery; LC = left cir-
cumflex coronary artery; P = posterior (noncoronary) cusp. Reproduced with permission of Lippincott-Raven
Publishers from Maron, B.J. *Heart disease and other cardiovascular risks in competitive athletes.* In:
Cardiology. Parmley, W.W., Chatterje, K. (Eds.). 1997, 3: 1-19.

Patients with anomalous left main coronary from the right sinus of Valsalva, may die
suddenly as the first manifestation of their disease (usually under age 35) and about one-
third may experience premonitory symptoms such as angina or syncope or even acute

myocardial infarction, with the vast majority of these events related to exertion (34, 37, 40, 41). Indeed, occurrence of one or more episodes of exertional syncope in a young athlete should require the definitive exclusion of coronary anomalies. Also, in youthful athletes it may be possible to raise a strong suspicion of (or even identify) anomalous left main coronary artery with conventional cross-sectional, two-dimensional or trans-esophageal echocardiography (42-46), leading to definitive confirmation by coronary arteriography. These considerations are particularly important because coronary anomalies, while rarely identified during life, are nevertheless amenable to corrective surgery.

The mechanism by which this coronary anomaly produces sudden death or syncope remains unresolved (34, 37, 40). Indeed, the presumably episodic nature of these events contributes substantially to this uncertainty. Several potential mechanisms have been put forward to explain myocardial ischemia and sudden death due to critical and sporadic impairment of coronary flow in patients with wrong sinus coronary anomalies (34, 37, 40, 41): the acute angle take-off and kinking of the coronary artery as it arises from the aorta; flap-like closure of the abnormal slit-like coronary orifice; compression of the anomalous coronary artery between the aorta and pulmonary trunk during exercise; and spasm of the anomalous coronary artery possibly due to endothelial injury. In some patients, the proximal portion of the anomalous coronary artery is essentially intramural (*i.e.*, within the aortic tunica media), which can further aggravate the coronary obstruction, particularly with expansion of the aorta during exercise.

Roberts *et al.* (35-37) emphasized that the "mirror image" coronary anomaly in which the *right* coronary artery arises from the *left* sinus of Valsalva (coursing between aorta and pulmonary trunk) may also convey risk for sudden death in young individuals (Fig. 4). With this lesion, an anatomical and pathophysiological situation exits at the right coronary ostium which is analogous to that previously described for the left main ostium when that artery originates from the right sinus. Presumably, the mechanism by which myocardial ischemia occurs in these two anatomic variants is similar.

MYOCARDITIS

Usually of acquired viral etiology, myocarditis has been considered an important cause of sudden unexplained death in young individuals (18, 47, 48). Myocarditis can occur in this context, often with no or relatively innocent prodromal symptoms, and definitive diagnosis may be difficult clinically as well as at necropsy (particularly in the healed phase). The importance of myocarditis as a cause of sudden death in the young may well have been exaggerated previously due to overinterpretation of histological data and the lack of standardized morphological criteria (49); however, others have maintained that this diagnosis is often overlooked (48).

In a large autopsy series of 134 competitive athletes, four (or 3%) showed areas of myocardium with acute inflammatory changes consisting of mononuclear cell infiltration associated with myocyte necrosis, consistent with myocarditis (Fig. 5) (1), whereas four other athletes showed areas of idiopathic myocardial scarring conceivably representing the healed phase of myocarditis. Of note, in the two high visibility tragedies concerning competitive athletes with cardiovascular disease in the United States – Hank Gathers and Reggie Lewis – the clinical and pathological findings were most consistent with myocarditis (50). While myocarditis in athletes is usually triggered by a viral infection, other etiologies such as chronic cocaine abuse can result in a similar clinical and pathologic profile (51-53).

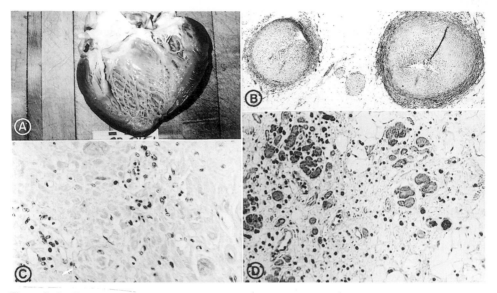

Figure 5. Cardiac morphological findings at autopsy in four competitive athletes who died suddenly. A: gross specimen from an athlete with greatly enlarged ventricular cavities, consistent with dilated cardiomyopathy. B: histological section of the left anterior descending coronary artery (left) and a diagonal branch (right) showing severe (>95%) cross-sectional luminal narrowing by atherosclerotic plaque. C: foci of inflammatory cells consistent with myocarditis. D: histological section of right ventricular wall showing islands of myocytes within a matrix of fatty and fibrous replacement, characteristic of arrhythmogenic right ventricular cardiomyopathy. Adapted from (1) with the permission of American Medical Association.

INTRAMURAL CORONARY ARTERY

It has also been suggested periodically that major coronary arteries "tunnelled" within left ventricular myocardium (*i.e.*, myocardial bridging) constitute a potentially lethal anatomic variant that may cause sudden unexpected death in otherwise healthy young individuals during exertion or stress (54-57). Such coronary arterial bridging (usually involving the left anterior descending) are completely surrounded by myocardium for at least a portion of their course (about 1-3 cm). It has been postulated that when certain susceptible individuals are subjected to a critical degree of systolic arterial compression, myocardial ischemia may result, even in the absence of hemodynamically significant atherosclerotic disease (and despite the fact that most coronary flow occurs in diastole) (37). Indeed, in about 5% of our of athletic field deaths a tunnelled left anterior descending coronary artery was present in the *absence* of any other structural anomaly (1). A clinical report in patients with myocardial bridges showed that the administration of short-acting beta-blockers during atrial pacing alleviated anginal symptoms and signs of ischemia by normalizing flow velocities and increasing luminal diameter of the tunnelled segments, supporting the view that tunnelled arteries may be of pathophysiological significance (56, 57). Most recently, myocardial ischemia produced by systolic compression of the left anterior descending coronary artery has been incriminated as a primary cause of sudden death in young patients with HCM (57).

AORTIC RUPTURE (AND MARFAN'S SYNDROME)
Marfan's syndrome is a particularly rare disease entity and an uncommon cause of sudden death in athletes due to aortic dissection and/or rupture (1, 5, 8, 9). Some such individuals may have the classic physical stigmata of Marfan's syndrome, although others may not. Individuals with Marfan's syndrome may participate successfully in strenuous competitive sports for many years, presumably prior to the time aortic dilatation becomes marked and a predisposition for dissection or rupture increases critically (Fig. 6). Indeed, the presence or absence of aortic dilatation is the primary determinant of whether individuals with Marfan's syndrome should be judged medically eligible for intense athletic competition.

CORONARY ARTERY DISEASE
Atherosclerotic coronary artery disease is cited as an important cause for sudden death in youthful athletes in several reports (Fig. 5) (1-3, 58). However, Corrado *et al.* (58) and Burke *et al.* (3) have emphasized the occurrence of premature atherosclerotic coronary disease as a common cause of sudden death in young people (including athletes) in the

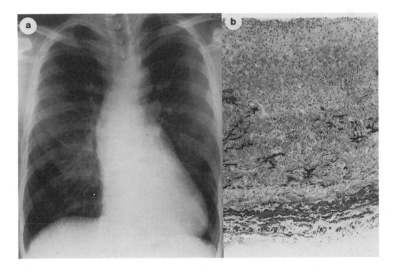

Figure 6. Marfan's syndrome. A: posteroanterior chest radiograph obtained from an 18-year-old male collegiate swimmer who died 2 months later of a ruptured aorta during a training session. Prominent dilatation of the ascending aorta is apparent, which was confirmed with echocardiography. In this patient, the correct diagnosis was made during life and the athlete was advised of (but ignored) the risks of continued competition. B: histological section of ascending aorta from another athlete who died of a ruptured aorta. Note the markedly diminished number of darkly stained elastic fibers in the aortic media. Intima is to the top and adventitia is to the bottom. Elastic van Gieson stain; x80. Reproduced from (5) with the permission of the American Heart Association.

United States and in the Veneto Region of northeastern Italy, respectively. Sudden death related to physical exertion, in the presence of severe coronary artery disease, is associated with acute plaque rupture (59).

VALVULAR HEART DISEASE

Aortic valvular stenosis had previously been regarded to be a common cause of sudden death in children and young asymptomatic adults, based on data from hospital-based populations (47). However, aortic stenosis is only occasionally an explanation for sudden death in young athletes. This is probably due to the fact that this lesion is likely to be identified early in life by virtue of the characteristically loud heart murmur, ultimately leading to disqualification from organized sports (60).

Despite its relative frequency in the general population (probably about 5%), mitral valve prolapse (61, 62) has not proved to be an important cause of sudden death in competitive sports. To date, only about 100 individuals with mitral prolapse have been reported to have died suddenly (average age about 35 years), rarely related to intense physical exertion or sporting activity, and reportedly occurring (to date) in less than five young trained athletes (18).

CARDIAC CONDUCTION SYSTEM ABNORMALITIES

Some authors (5, 9, 63-66) have suggested that a spectrum of occult abnormalities in the cardiac conduction system (in the absence of other structural cardiac abnormalities) may be responsible for sudden death in competitive athletes and other young people with otherwise structurally normal hearts. For example, Thiene et al. (65) reported three young athletes with a variety of atrioventricular conduction system abnormalities, including one with accessory atrioventricular pathways. James et al. (66) and Burke et al. (63) described morphological abnormalities of the small intramural artery to the sinoatrial node, consisting of thickened vessel wall and narrowed lumen which they incriminated as the determinant of degeneration, scarring and hemorrhage present in the surrounding conducting tissue, and the cause of sudden death.

ARRHYTHMOGENIC RIGHT VENTRICULAR CARDIOMYOPATHY

Arrhythmogenic right ventricular cardiomyopathy (ARVC) is an unusual and often familial condition associated with important ventricular or supraventricular arrhythmias, which has also been cited as a cause of sudden death in the young (including athletes) (67-72). ARVC is characterized morphologically by myocyte death in the right ventricular wall with replacement fibrous and/or adipose tissue formation as evidence of repair, often associated with myocarditis and apoptosis (Fig. 5). This right ventricular disease process may be diffuse or, alternatively, segmental and involve only limited portions of the wall.

Investigators in northeastern Italy have reported ARVC to be the most common cause of sudden death in young athletes. The relatively frequent occurrence of ARVC in this particular region of Italy may reflect a unique genetic substrate. Furthermore, the low frequency with which HCM is apparently responsible for sudden death in Italian athletes is an interesting, but also largely unresolved issue. It is possible that the long-standing and systematic Italian national program for the cardiovascular assessment of competitive athletes (73) has had the effect of identifying and disqualifying disproportionate numbers of trained athletes with HCM, due to the fact that this cardiac disease is more easily identifiable clinically than ARVC (69).

ABSENCE OF APPARENT STRUCTURAL DISEASE

Occasional athletes dying suddenly demonstrate no evidence of structural cardiovascular disease, even after careful gross and microscopic examination of the heart (1). In such instances (about 2% of our series) (1) it may not be possible to exclude with certainty noncardiac factors (such as drug abuse), or occult but clinically relevant abnormalities of the specialized conducting system and associated vasculature (63-66). It is also possible that such deaths are due to rare conditions in which structural abnormalities of the heart are characteristically lacking at necropsy such as long QT syndrome (26, 74, 75), primary ventricular fibrillation (76, 77), or unrecognized segmental ARVC or previously unidentified Wolff-Parkinson-White syndrome. There is no evidence at present that systemic hypertension, per se, is associated with increased risk for sudden cardiac death in young athletes (78).

Sudden Cardiac Death in Older Trained Athletes

Increasing numbers of middle-aged or older individuals are now participating in organized competitive sports and vigorous physical conditioning programs. However, superior physical fitness in this age group (or at any other age) does not guarantee protection against exercise-related death in the presence of underlying cardiovascular disease. As is the case with the young competitive athlete, older athletes may harbor occult cardiac disease and die suddenly and unexpectedly while participating in athletic activities (9-15). Nevertheless, the incidence of such catastrophes (and therefore the risk) is quite low considering the large number of individuals participating in sporting activities (11, 13).

Unlike youthful athletes, the cause of death in older conditioned athletes (age >35) is usually not a congenital malformation of the heart, but atherosclerotic coronary artery disease in the vast majority of instances (Fig. 7). The remaining deaths in older athletes are due to a variety of noncoronary etiologies, such as valvular heart disease, including mitral valve prolapse, or HCM (9, 79).

Older trained athletes who have died suddenly during or just following physical activity of coronary heart disease comprise a heterogeneous athletic population including runners training for competitive long distance races and joggers, as well as participants in sports such as rugby and squash. In contrast to young competitive athletes with congenital heart disease, over one-half of the older athletes with coronary heart disease had either experienced prodromal cardiovascular symptoms, had knowledge of their underlying disease, or specific documentation of prior myocardial infarction.

Mechanisms and Resuscitation

Although the precise mechanism ultimately responsible for sudden death in young athletes depends on the particular disease state involved, in the vast majority of instances

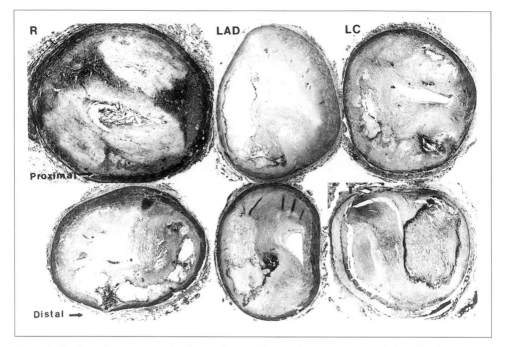

Figure 7. Sections of coronary arteries from a 49-year-old man who ran an average of about 170 km per week and successfully completed six marathons and seven 80 km races, but died suddenly of coronary heart disease. The right (R), left anterior descending (LAD) and left circumflex (LC) coronary arteries are shown at the sites of maximal narrowing by atherosclerosis, both in the proximal (upper panels) and distal (lower panels) halves of the respective arteries. Reproduced from (9) with the permission of the Journal of American College of Cardiology.

cardiac arrest results from electrical instability and ventricular tachyarrhythmias. In the case of HCM, the disorganized cardiac muscle cells distributed widely throughout the left ventricular wall probably represent the substrate for ventricular tachycardia/fibrillation when associated with a number of potential clinical triggers (including intense physical activity) (Fig. 8) (80). A clear exception to this model is Marfan's syndrome in which sudden death is due to aortic rupture. Of note, regardless of the underlying mechanism, very few athletes with cardiovascular disease who collapse on the athletic field are successfully resuscitated.

It is possible that the routine presence of automatic external defibrillators at athletic events (and public access defibrillation) would lead to the survival of greater numbers of such athletes (81). However, the great infrequency with which these events occur ultimately represents an obstacle to efficient resuscitation practice on the rare occasion of such an event. Therefore, it would appear equally important to emphasize the early detection of potentially lethal cardiovascular abnormalities through preparticipation screening (60) and the withdrawal of such athletes from intense training and competition (17).

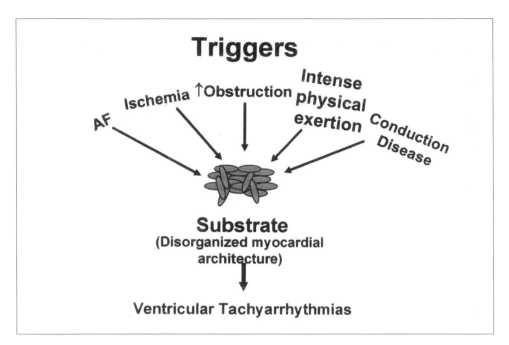

Figure 8. Proposed mechanisms by which sudden cardiac death may occur in athletes with hypertrophic cardiomyopathy. AF = atrial fibrillation.

Eligibility Considerations for Athletes with Known Cardiovascular Disease

When a cardiovascular abnormality is identified in a young competitive athlete two important considerations arise: i) the magnitude of risk for sudden cardiac death associated with continued participation in competitive sports; and ii) the criteria to be implemented for determining whether recommendations for withdrawal from sports competition are appropriate for a given athlete. In this regard, the 26th Bethesda Conference sponsored by the American College of Cardiology (17) in 1994 offered prospective and consensus recommendations for athletic eligibility or disqualification, by taking into account the nature and severity of the cardiovascular abnormality as well as the type and level of sports training and competition (Fig. 9). The 26th Bethesda Conference recommendations (17) were predicated on the likelihood that intense athletic training will increase the risk for sudden cardiac death (or disease progression) in trained athletes with clinically important structural heart disease. Although at present it is not possible to quantify that risk with precision for the many cardiac diseases involved, it is a reasonable assumption that the temporary or permanent withdrawal of selected athletes from participation in certain intense competitive sports is both prudent and beneficial by virtue of mitigating the perceived risk for sudden death (82).

These considerations are particularly relevant to a heterogeneous disease such as HCM, in which risk stratification remains incompletely precise (21, 23). The fact that it is difficult to stratify risk for individual athletes (or patients) with HCM is reflected in the

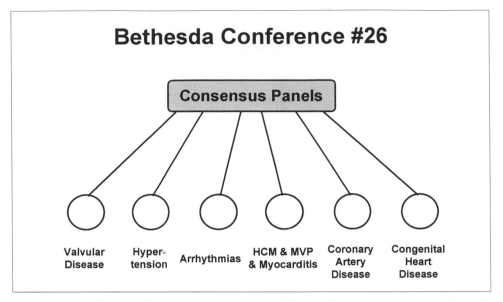

Figure 9. Format of Bethesda Conference #26 consensus panel (17), providing recommendations for athletic eligibility or disqualification for over 70 cardiovascular abnormalities or diseases, and with respect to the level and intensity of athletic training and competition. HCM = hypertrophic cardiomyopathy; MVP = mitral valve prolapse.

26th Bethesda Conference recommendations (17) for athletic eligibility that are necessarily conservative and homogeneous for most athletes with HCM. Indeed, for HCM as well as other diseases with a propensity for potentially lethal arrhythmias, the stress of athletic training and competition as well as associated alterations in blood volume, hydration and electrolytes may in fact elevate the level of risk over that of a nonathlete with the same disease. This report (17) provided clear guidelines and benchmarks for the expected standards of care. Indeed, the Bethesda recommendations have recently been cited by the Court (in Knapp *vs.* Northwestern University) as a consensus reference document that the team physician should rely upon in formulating disqualification decisions for competitive athletes with cardiovascular disease (83).

> *"Death should stay away from young men's*
> *games. Death belongs in musty hospital rooms,*
> *sickbeds. It should not impinge its terrible*
> *presence on the celebrations of youth, reap its*
> *frightful harvest in fields where cheers ring and*
> *bands play and banners wave."*

Jim Murray

References

1. Maron, B.J., Shirani, J., Poliac, L.C. et al. *Sudden death in young competitive athletes: Clinical, demographic and pathological profiles.* JAMA 1996, 276: 199-204.
2. Van Camp, S.P., Bloor, C.M., Mueller, F.O. et al. *Nontraumatic sports death in high school and college athletes.* Med Sci Sports Exer 1995, 27: 641-7.
3. Burke, A.P., Farb, A., Virmani, R. et al. *Sports-related and non-sports-related sudden cardiac death in young athletes.* Am Heart J 1991, 121: 568-75.
4. Corrado, D., Thiene, G., Nava, A. et al. *Sudden death in young competitive athletes: Clinicopathologic correlations in 22 cases.* Am J Med 1990, 39: 588-96.
5. Maron, B.J., Roberts, W.C., McAllister, H.A. et al. *Sudden death in young athletes.* Circulation 1980, 62: 218-29.
6. Driscoll, D.J., Edwards, W.D. *Sudden unexpected death in children and adolescents.* J Am Coll Cardiol 1985, 5: 118B-21B.
7. Drory, Y., Turetz, Y., Hiss, Y. et al. *Sudden unexpected death in persons less than 40 years of age.* Am J Cardiol 1991, 68: 1388-92.
8. Liberthson, R.R. *Sudden death from cardiac causes in children and young adults.* N Engl J Med 1996, 334: 1039-44.
9. Maron, B.J., Epstein, S.E., Roberts, W.C. *Causes of sudden death in the competitive athlete.* J Am Coll Cardiol 1986, 7: 204-14.
10. Virmani, R., Robinowitz, M., McAllister, H.A. *Nontraumatic death in joggers. A series of 30 patients at autopsy.* Am J Med 1982, 72: 874-82.
11. Thompson, P.D., Funk, E.J., Carleton, R.A. et al. *Incidence of death during jogging in Rhode Island from 1975 through 1980.* JAMA 1982, 247: 2535-8.
12. Waller, B.F., Roberts, W.C. *Sudden death while running in conditioned runners aged 40 years or over.* Am J Cardiol 1980, 45: 1292-1300.
13. Maron, B.J., Poliac, L.C., Roberts, W.O. *Risk for sudden cardiac death associated with marathon running.* J Am Coll Cardiol 1996, 28: 428-31.
14. Opie, L.H. *Sudden death and sport.* Lancet 1985, 254: 1321-5.
15. Thompson, P.D., Stern, M.P., Williams, P. et al. *Death during jogging or running. A study of 18 cases.* JAMA 1979, 242: 1265-7.
16. Maron, B.J. *Sudden death in young athletes: Lessons from the Hank Gathers affair.* N Engl J Med 1993, 329: 55-7.
17. Maron, B.J., Mitchell, J.H. *26th Bethesda Conference. Recommendations for determining eligibility for competition in athletes with cardiovascular abnormalities.* J Am Coll Cardiol 1994, 24: 845-99.
18. Maron, B.J., Isner, J.M., McKenna, W.J. *Hypertrophic cardiomyopathy, myocarditis and other myopericardial diseases, and mitral valve prolapse. Task Force 3.* In: 26th Bethesda Conference. Recommendations for Determining Eligibility for Competition in Athletes with Cardiovascular Abnormalities (BJ Maron and JH Mitchell). J Am Coll Cardiol 1994, 24: 880-5.
19. Maron, B.J., Bonow, R.O., Cannon, R.O. et al. *Hypertrophic cardiomyopathy: Interrelation of clinical manifestations, pathophysiology, and therapy.* N Engl J Med 1987, 316: 780-89, 844-52.
20. Wigle, E.D., Sasson, Z., Henderson, M.A. et al. *Hypertrophic cardiomyopathy. The importance of the site and extent of hypertrophy. A review.* Prog Cardiovasc Dis 1985, 28: 1-83.
21. Spirito, P., Seidman, C.E., McKenna, S.J., Maron, B.J. *The management of hypertrophic cardiomyopathy.* N Engl J Med 1997, 36: 775-85.
22. Klues, H.G., Schiffers, A., Maron, B.J. *Phenotypic spectrum and patterns of left ventricular hypertrophy in hypertrophic cardiomyopathy: Morphologic observations and significance as assessed by two-dimensional echocardiography in 600 patients.* J Am Coll Cardiol 1995, 26: 1699-1708.
23. Maron, B.J. *Hypertrophic cardiomyopathy.* Lancet 1997, 350: 127-33.
24. Maron, B.J. *Hypertrophic cardiomyopathy.* Curr Probl Cardiol 1993, 18: 643-704.
25. Maron, B.J., Gardin, J.M., Flack, J.M. et al. *Assessment of the prevalence of hypertrophic cardiomyopathy in a general population of young adults: Echocardiographic analysis of 4111 subjects in the CARDIA study.* Circulation 1995, 92: 785-9.

26. Maron, B.J., Moller, J.H., Seidman, C.E. et al. *Impact of laboratory molecular diagnosis on contemporary diagnostic criteria for genetically transmitted cardiovascular diseases: Hypertrophic cardiomyopathy, long-QT syndrome, and Marfan syndrome.* Circulation 1998, 98: 1460-71.

27. Maron, B.J., Roberts, W.C., Epstein, S.E. *Sudden death in hypertrophic cardiomyopathy: A profile of 78 patients.* Circulation 1982, 65: 1388-94.

28. Maron, B.J., Klues, H.G. *Surviving competitive athletics with hypertrophic cardiomyopathy.* Am J Cardiol 1994, 73: 1098-1104.

29. Maron, B.J., Epstein, S.E. *Hypertrophic cardiomyopathy: A discussion of nomenclature.* Am J Cardiol 1979, 43: 1242-4.

30. Maron, B.J., Gottdiener, J.S., Epstein, S.E. *Patterns and significance of the distribution of left ventricular hypertrophy in hypertrophic cardiomyopathy: A wide-angle, two-dimensional echocardiographic study of 125 patients.* Am J Cardiol 1981, 48: 418-28.

31. Maron, B.J., Gross, B.W., Stark, S.I. *Extreme left ventricular hypertrophy.* Circulation 1995, 92: 3748.

32. Niimura, H., Bachinski, L.L., Sangwatanaorj, S. et al. *Human cardiac myosin-binding protein C and late-onset familial hypertrophic cardiomyopathy.* N Engl J Med 1998, 338: 1248-57.

33. Charron, P., Dubourg, O., Desnos, M. et al. *Diagnostic value of electrocardiography and echocardiography for familial hypertrophic cardiomyopathy in a genotyped adult population.* Circulation 1997, 96: 214-19.

34. Cheitlin, M.D., De Castro, C.M., McAllister, H.A. *Sudden death as a complication of anomalous left coronary origin from the anterior sinus of Valsalva, a not-so-minor congenital anomaly.* Circulation 1974, 50: 780-7.

35. Roberts, W.C., Kragel, A.H. *Anomalous origin of either the right or left main coronary artery from the aorta with subsequent coursing of the anomalously arising artery between aorta and pulmonary trunk.* Am J Cardiol 1988, 62: 1263-7.

36. Kragel, A.H., Roberts, W.C. *Anomalous origin of either the right or left main coronary artery from the aorta with subsequent coursing between aorta and pulmonary trunk: Analysis of 32 necropsy cases.* Am J Cardiol 1988, 62: 771-7.

37. Roberts, W.C. *Congenital coronary arterial anomalies unassociated with major anomalies of the heart or great vessels.* In: Adult Congenital Heart Disease. Roberts, W.C. (Ed.). FA Davis Co.: Philadelphia 1987: 583-629.

38. Taylor, A.J., Rogan, K.M., Virmani, R. *Sudden cardiac death associated with isolated congenital coronary artery anomalies.* J Am Coll Cardiol 1992, 20: 640-7.

39. Virmani, R., Chun, P.K.C., Goldstein, R.E. et al. *Acute takeoffs of the coronary arteries along the aortic wall and congenital coronary ostial valve-like ridges: Association with sudden death.* J Am Coll Cardiol 1984, 3: 766-71.

40. Chaitman, B.R., Lespérance, J., Saltiel, J. et al. *Clinical, angiographic, and hemodynamic findings in patients with anomalous origin of the coronary arteries.* Circulation 1976, 53: 122-31.

41. Basso, C., Maron, B.J., Corrado, D., Thiene, G. *Clinical profile of congenital coronary artery anomalies with origin from the wrong aortic sinus leading to sudden death in young competitive athletes (abstract).* Circulation 1998, 98 (Suppl I): 1-618.

42. Maron, B.J., Leon, M.B., Swain, J.A. et al. *Prospective identification by two-dimensional echocardiography of anomalous origin of the left main coronary artery from the right sinus of Valsalva.* Am J Cardiol 1991, 68: 140-2.

43. Jureidini, S.B., Eaton, C., Williams, J. et al. *Transthoracic two-dimensional and color flow echocardiographic diagnosis of aberrant left coronary artery.* Am Heart J 1994, 127: 438-40.

44. Salloum, J.A., Thomas, D., Evans, J. *Transesophageal echocardiography in diagnosis of aberrant coronary artery.* Int J Cardiol 1991, 32: 106-8.

45. Alam, M., Brymer, J., Smith, S. *Transesophageal echocardiographic diagnosis of anomalous left coronary artery from the right aortic sinus.* Chest 1993, 103: 1617-18.

46. Gaither, N.S., Rogan, K.M., Stajduhr, K. et al. *Anomalous origin and course of coronary arteries in adults: Identification and improved imaging utilizing transesophageal echocardiography.* Am Heart J 1991, 122: 69-75.

47. Lambert, E.C., Menon, V.A., Wagner, H.R. et al. *Sudden unexpected death from cardiovascular disease in children. A cooperative international study.* Am J Cardiol 1974, 34: 89-96.

48. Wesslen, L., Pahlson, C., Lindquist, O. et al. *An increase in sudden unexpected cardiac deaths among young Swedish orienteers during 1979-1992.* Eur Heart J 1996, 17: 902-10.

49. Aretz, H.T., Billingham, M.E., Edwards, W.D. et al. *Myocarditis. A histopathologic definition and classification.* Am J Cardiovasc Pathol 1986, 1: 3-14.

50. Maron, B.J., Garson, A. *Arrhythmias and sudden cardiac death in elite athletes.* Cardiol Rev 1994, 2(1): 26-32.

51. Isner, J.M., Estes, N.A.M. III, Thompson, P.D. et al. *Acute cardiac events temporally related to cocaine abuse.* N Engl J Med 1986, 315: 1438-43.

52. Kloner, R.A., Hale, S., Alkekr, K. et al. *The effects of acute and chronic cocaine use on the heart.* Circulation 1992, 85: 407-19.

53. Virmani, R., Robinowitz, M., Smialek, J.E. et al. *Cardiovascular effects of cocaine: An autopsy study of 40 patients.* Am Heart J 1988, 115: 1068-76.

54. Morales, A.R., Romanelli, R., Boucek, R.J. *The mural left anterior descending coronary artery, strenuous exercise and sudden death.* Circulation 1980, 62: 230-7.

55. Noble, J., Bourassa, M.G., Petitclerc, R. *Myocardial bridging and milking effect of the left anterior descending coronary artery: Normal variant or obstruction?* Am J Cardiol 1976, 37: 993-9.

56. Schwarz, E.R., Klues, H.G., vom Dahl, J. et al. *Functional, angiographic and intracoronary Doppler flow characteristics in symptomatic patients with myocardial bridging: Effect of short-term intravenous beta-blocker medication.* J Am Coll Cardiol 1996, 27: 1637-45.

57. Yetman, A.T., McCrindle, B.W., MacDonald, C., Freedom, R.M., Gow, R. *Myocardial bridging in children with hypertrophic cardiomyopathy - a risk factor for sudden death.* N Engl J Med 1998, 339: 1201-9.

58. Corrado, D., Basso, C., Poletti, A. et al. *Sudden death in the young. Is acute coronary thrombosis the major precipitating factor?* Circulation 1994, 90: 2315-23.

59. Burke, A.P., Farb, A., Malcom, G.T., Liang, Y.-H., Smialek, J.E., Virmani, R. *Plaque rupture and sudden death related to exertion in men with coronary artery disease.* JAMA 1999, 281, 921-6.

60. Maron, B.J., Thompson, P.D., Puffer, J.C. et al. *Cardiovascular preparticipation screening of competitive athletes.* Circulation 1996, 94: 850-6.

61. Dollar, A.L., Roberts, W.C. *Morphologic comparison of patients with mitral valve prolapse who died suddenly with patients who died from severe valvular dysfunction or other conditions.* J Am Coll Cardiol 1991, 17: 921-31.

62. Chesler, E., King, R.A., Edwards, J.E. *The myxomatous mitral valve and sudden death.* Circulation 1983, 67: 632-9.

63. Burke, A.P., Subramanian, R., Smialek, J. et al. *Nonatherosclerotic narrowing of the atrioventricular node artery and sudden death.* J Am Coll Cardiol 1993, 21: 117-22.

64. Corrado, D., Thiene, G., Cocco, P., Frescura, C. *Non-atherosclerotic coronary artery disease and sudden death in the young.* Br Heart J 1992, 68: 601-7.

65. Thiene, G., Pennelli, N., Rossi, L. *Cardiac conduction system abnormalities as a possible cause of sudden death in young athletes.* Human Pathol 1983, 14: 706-9.

66. James, T.N., Froggatt, P., Marshall, T.K. *Sudden death in young athletes.* Ann Int Med 1967, 67: 1013-21.

67. Thiene, G., Nava, A., Corrado, D. et al. *Right ventricular cardiomyopathy and sudden death in young people.* N Engl J Med 1988, 318: 129-33.

68. Furlanello, F., Bertoldi, A., Dallago, M. et al. *Cardiac arrest and sudden death in competitive athletes with arrhythmogenic right ventricular dysplasia.* PACE 1998, 21: 331-5.

69. McKenna, W.J., Thiene, G., Nava, A. et al. *Diagnosis of arrhythmogenic right ventricular dysplasia/cardiomyopathy.* Br Heart J 1994, 71: 215-18.

70. Basso, C., Thiene, G., Corrado, D. et al. *Arrhythmogenic right ventricular cardiomyopathy: Dysplasia, dystrophy or myocarditis?* Circulation 1996, 94: 983-91.

71. Daliento, L., Turrini, P., Nava, A. et al. *Arrhythmogenic right ventricular cardiomyopathy in young versus adult patients: Similarities and differences.* J Am Coll Cardiol 1995, 25: 655-64.

72. Corrado, D., Basso, C., Thiene, G. et al. *Spectrum of clinicopathologic manifestations of arrhythmogenic right ventricular cardiomyopathy/dysplasia: A multicenter study.* J Am Coll Cardiol 1997, 30: 1512-20.

73. Pelliccia, A., Maron, B.J. *Preparticipation cardiovascular evaluation of the competitive athlete: Perspectives from the 30 year Italian experience.* Am J Cardiol 1995, 75: 827-8.

74. Vincent, C.M., Timothy, K.W., Leppert, M. et al. *The spectrum of symptoms and QT intervals in carriers of the gene for the long-QT syndrome.* N Engl J Med 1992, 327: 846-52.

75. Moss, A.J., Schwartz, P.J., Crampton, R.S. et al. *The long QT syndrome: Prospective longitudinal study of 328 families.* Circulation 1991, 84: 1136-44.

76. Benson, D.W., Benditt, D.G., Anderson, R.W. et al. *Cardiac arrest in young, ostensibly healthy patients: Clinical, hemodynamic and electrophysiologic findings.* Am J Cardiol 1983, 52: 65-9.

77. Fan, W., Peter, C.T. *Survival and incidence of appropriate shocks in implantable cardioverter defibrillator recipients who have no detectable structural heart disease.* Am J Cardiol 1994, 74: 687-90.

78. Kaplan, N.M., Deveraux, R.B., Miller, H.S., Jr. *26th Bethesda Conference: Recommendations for determining eligibility for competition in athletes with cardiovascular abnormalities. Task Force 4: Systemic hypertension.* J Am Coll Cardiol 1994, 24: 885-8.

79. Noakes, T.D., Rose, A.G., Opie, L.H. *Hypertrophic cardiomyopathy associated with sudden death during marathon racing.* Br Heart J 1979, 41: 624-7.

80. Maron, B.J., Roberts, W.C. *Quantitative analysis of cardiac muscle cell disorganization in the ventricular septum of patients with hypertrophic cardiomyopathy.* Circulation 1979, 59: 689-706.

81. Kerber, R.E., Becker, L.B., Bourland, J.D. et al. *Automatic external defibrillators for public access defibrillation: Recommendations for specifying and reporting arrhythmia analysis algorithm performance, incorporating new waveforms, and enhancing safety.* Circulation 1997, 95: 1677-82.

82. Corrado, D., Basso, C., Schiavon, M., Thiene G. *Screening for hypertrophic cardiomyopathy in young athletes.* N Engl J Med 1998, 339: 364-9.

83. Maron, B.J., Mitten, M.J., Quandt, E.K., Zipes D.P. *Competitive athletes with cardiovascular disease - the case of Nicholas Knapp.* N Engl J Med 1998, 339: 1632-5.

CHAPTER 5

PATHOLOGY OF SUDDEN DEATH IN YOUNG ATHLETES:
THE EUROPEAN EXPERIENCE

G. Thiene, C. Basso and D. Corrado
*Institute of Pathological Anatomy, University of Padua Medical School,
Padua, Italy*

Introduction

For centuries it was a mystery why cardiac arrest should occur in young vigorous athletes, who had previously achieved extraordinary exercise performance without complaining of any symptoms. The cause was generally ascribed to myocardial infarction, even though evidence of regional ischemic myocyte necrosis had rarely been reported. It is now clear that the usual mechanism is an abrupt arrhythmia, that a wide spectrum of cardiovascular abnormalities may cause sudden death in young athletes and that even minor lesions may be life-threatening by jeopardizing the electrical order of the heart during effort (1-16). The culprit diseases are clinically covert and unlikely to be diagnosed or suspected. Early identification might reduce the risk and incidence of sudden death and systematic preparticipation screening for qualification of individuals embarking in competitive sports is now carried out in some countries such as Italy. However, the efficacy and cost-effectiveness of this screening is the subject of debate.

In this paper, we will review the prevalence, morbid causes and mechanisms of sudden death in athletes and compare the medical examination of athletes in North America and Italy in order to assess whether the rigorous Italian protocol is able to prevent sudden death.

Prevalence of Sudden Death in Young Athletes: The Experience of the Veneto Region

Forty-nine young athletes died suddenly in the Veneto Region between 1979 and 1996 (17). They were part of 269 sudden deaths in the young (≤ 35 years) that were studied in the same time period. The prevalence of sudden death was calculated as 0.75/100,000/year among young nonathletes (sudden infant death excluded) and 1.6/100,000 among young athletes ($p < 0.01$). The overall prevalence in the young was calculated as 0.8/100,000/year. The higher percentage in athletes clearly demonstrates the role of strenuous exercise in increasing the risk of sudden death.

Table 1 shows the spectrum of diseases accounting for sudden death in young athletes and nonathletes. Cardiovascular diseases are by far the leading cause.

Among nonathletes, atherosclerotic coronary artery disease ranks first on the list, followed by mitral valve prolapse, conduction system disease, myocarditis, arrhythmogenic

49

A. Bayés de Luna et al. (eds.), Arrhythmias and Sudden Death in Athletes, 49–69.
© 2000 *Kluwer Academic Publishers. Printed in the Netherlands.*

right ventricular cardiomyopathy, hypertrophic cardiomyopathy and aortic dissection. Among athletes, arrhythmogenic right ventricular cardiomyopathy ranks first, followed by atherosclerotic coronary artery diseases, congenital coronary anomalies and mitral valve prolapse.

Table 1. Causes of sudden death in athletes and nonathletes 35 years of age or less in the Veneto region of Italy from 1979 to 1996. Reproduced with permission from (17).

Cause	Total	Athletes	Nonathletes
Arrhythmogenic right ventricular cardiomyopathy	29 (10.8%)	11 (22.4%)	18 (8.2%)*
Atherosclerotic coronary artery disease	45 (16.7%)	9 (18.4%)	36 (16.4%)
Anomalous origin of coronary artery	7 (2.6%)	6 (12.2%)	1 (0.5%)
Disease of conduction system	24 (8.9%)	4 (8.2%)	20 (9.1%)
Mitral valve prolapse	26 (9.7%)	5 (10.2%)	21 (9.5%)
Hypertrophic cardiomyopathy	17 (6.3%)	1 (2.0%)	16 (7.3%)
Myocarditis	22 (8.2%)	3 (6.1%)	19 (8.6%)
Myocardial bridge	7 (2.6%)	2 (4.1%)	5 (2.3%)
Pulmonary thromboembolism	4 (1.5%)	1 (2.0%)	3 (1.4%)
Dissecting aortic aneurysm	12 (4.5%)	1 (2.0%)	11 (5.0%)
Dilated cardiomyopathy	10 (3.7%)	1 (2.0%)	9 (4.1%)
Other	66 (24.5%)	5 (10.2%)	61 (27.7%)
Total	269	49	220

$p = 0.008$ for the comparison with the athletes; *$p <0.001$ for the comparison with the athletes.

When the various diseases were compared, only arrhythmogenic right ventricular cardiomyopathy and congenital anomalies of coronary arteries occurred more frequently in athletes than in nonathletes (22.4% *vs.* 8.2% and 12.2% *vs.* 0.5%, respectively), which indicates that these diseases are particularly likely to cause cardiac arrest during effort. Sudden deaths due to other diseases, such as atherosclerotic coronary artery disease, Wolff-Parkinson-White syndrome, mitral valve prolapse and myocarditis also occur, regardless of rest or exercise. On the other hand, hypertrophic cardiomyopathy, the most frequent cause of sudden death among athletes in North America (3, 6, 10, 11), occurred three times more frequently among nonathletes. Easy identification of affected subjects at preparticipation screening and subsequent disqualification may account for there being fewer athletes affected by hypertrophic cardiomyopathy exposed to the risk of sudden death during sport (17).

Table 2 shows the prodromic signs and symptoms of athletes who died suddenly due to the three major cardiovascular conditions, namely: arrhythmogenic right ventricular cardiomyopathy (n = 11), atherosclerotic coronary artery disease (n = 9) and congenital coronary artery anomalies (n = 8). The rarity of prodroma in patients affected by both acquired and congenital coronary artery disease, particularly the absence of chest pain, highlights the difficulty of suspecting these lesions. On the other hand, most patients with arrhythmogenic right ventricular cardiomyopathy had something that might have alerted them, either in terms of a family history of sudden death or in terms of electrical disorders (palpitations, syncope, electrocardiogram (ECG) abnormalities such as ST-T changes and arrhythmias).

Table 2. *Clinical findings at preparticipation screening of athletes who died suddenly of one of the leading three cardiovascular causes 1996. Reproduced with permission from (17).*

Findings	Cause of death		
	Arrhythmogenic right ventricular cardiomyopathy (n = 11)	Atherosclerotic coronary artery disease (n = 9)	Coronary artery anomaly* (n = 8)
Family history of sudden death from heart disease	2	0	0
Palpitations on exertion	6	1	0
Syncope	5	1	1
Chest pain	0	0	0
ST-segment or T-wave abnormalities	9	0	1
Ventricular arrhythmias	6	0	2
One or more of the above	9 (82%)	2 (22%)**	2 (25%)**

*This group includes both patients with anomalous origin of a coronary artery and those with myocardial bridges. **$p = 0.02$ for the comparison with those with arrhythmogenic right ventricular cardiomyopathy.

Mechanisms and Pathology of Sudden Death in Athletes

Extracardiac causes of sudden death are extremely rare in the athlete. By extracardiac causes we mean cerebral death due to stroke or apoplexy (for instance, spontaneous rupture of berry aneurysm) or respiratory failure (sudden ventilatory failure due to allergic asthma). In our experience, only one subarachnoid hemorrhage due to a ruptured berry aneurysm of the middle cerebral artery was observed in a young rugby player. Most cases of sudden death were cardiovascular in origin (17). The mechanism was mechanical either due to spontaneous aortic rupture and cardiac tamponade (one case) or to pulmonary thromboembolism (one case). In the remaining subjects, cardiac arrest was the result of an arrhythmic event, most probably ventricular fibrillation, in the setting of coronary artery disease, cardiomyopathies and myocarditis, conduction system abnormalities and mitral valve prolapse.

Atherosclerotic Coronary Artery Disease

This is the most common cause of exercise-related sudden death in adult and elderly subjects. Severe multivessel atherosclerotic coronary artery diseases, frequently associated with postinfarction scars and even coronary thrombosis with acute myocardial infarction, are the usual findings in joggers and marathon runners over 35 years of age who die suddenly (1-48). With these pathological substrates, pathophysiologic mechanisms of cardiac arrest include either primary ventricular arrhythmias arising from myocardial scars or otherwise an acute ischemic electrical instability, which may be precipitated by an effort-increased myocardial oxygen demand or by a fresh occlusive thrombosis (19). Our experience of sudden death in young competitive athletes (⩽35 years) was quite different (17, 20, 21). The subjects had no history of angina pectoris or abnormal ECG finding, either at rest or during exercise (Fig. 1 A, B). Moreover, sudden death was mostly the first manifestation of the disease and rarely occurred during exercise. At autopsy we never observed cases with ischemic scars or acute, regional myocardial infarction. Coronary atherosclerosis was quite peculiar, presenting with a single obstructive plaque mostly involving the proximal left anterior descending coronary artery (Fig. 1C); focal signs of acute myocyte ischemic damage were detected in the anteroseptal myocardium. The plaque, which was rarely complicated by thrombosis, was mostly fibrous with superimposed smooth muscle cell intimal proliferation (so-called accelerated atherosclerosis) and a preserved tunica media (21). In summary, both clinical and morphologic features are consistent with a cardiac arrest precipitated by transient vasospastic myocardial ischemia. The absence of warning symptoms and the poor sensitivity of stress tests in disclosing myocardial ischemia render arduous the *in vivo* identification of young athletes at risk of ischemic cardiac arrest.

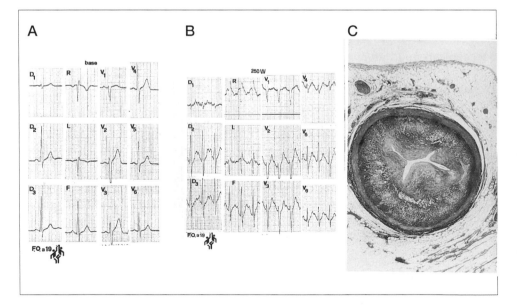

Figure 1. Sudden arrhythmic death due to atherosclerotic coronary artery disease in a 19-year-old basketball player. Both basal (A) and exercise test (B) electrocardiograms were normal. Nonetheless a severe concentric atherosclerotic plaque was evident in the proximal left anterior descending coronary artery (C): note the well-preserved tunica media (Heidenhain trichrome, o.m. original x 15).

Congenital Coronary Artery Anomalies

Congenital coronary artery anomalies, both of origin and course, are another leading cause of sudden death in young athletes (6, 7, 13, 14, 22, 23).

Apparently minor coronary artery malformations do exist, with an ostium located in a wrong aortic sinus, which have a silent clinical course and in which strenuous effort may precipitate ischemic cardiac arrest, obviously due to a discrepancy between coronary blood demand and supply. The congenital anomaly consists of both left and right coronary arteries arising from the same aortic sinus, whether left or right (Figs. 2, 3). In both conditions, the anomalous coronary artery arises from the aorta with an acute angle take-off and runs between the aorta and the pulmonary trunk, the first tract often disclosing an intramural course within the aortic tunica media. The coronary lumen shows a slit-like shape which, together with exercise-induced aortic root expansion and compression of the anomalous vessel against the pulmonary trunk, accounts for coronary blood flow shortage during sports performance. Anomalous origin of the left coronary artery from the right aortic sinus is considered more malignant than the right coronary artery from left aortic sinus (22). At postmortem examination the ventricular myocardium of the territory supplied by the anomalous coronary vessels may show acute or chronic ischemic damage (Fig. 2D). In two instances, an overt subacute, healed myocardial infarction was observed (24).

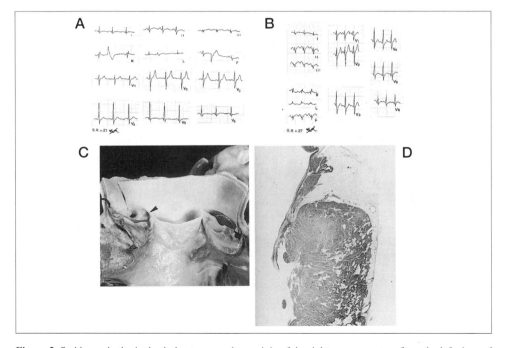

Figure 2. Sudden arrhythmic death due to anomalous origin of the right coronary artery from the left sinus of a 29-year-old rugby player. (A) Basal electrocardiogram shows a single premature ventricular beat. (B) Exercise stress test electrocardiogram is normal. (C) View of the aortic root showing the right coronary artery arising from the left sinus of Valsalva (arrow). (D) Extensive subepicardial posterior healed myocardial infarction at histologic section (Heidenhain trichrome, o.m. original x 3).

Unfortunately, the effort-related mechanisms of myocardial ischemia are difficult to reproduce in the clinical setting. Negative ECG was seen not only in basal conditions but also during exercise testing in young athletes with the above mentioned coronary anomalies who subsequently died suddenly during sports (Figs. 2 A, B). Chest pain may be absent in the history of these subjects, who may experience only atypical prodroma in the form of palpitation and/or syncope due to ventricular arrhythmias during effort. Thus, even if exercise testing is normal and there is no chest pain, an underlying ischemic substrate should be suspected in young athletes with apparently benign symptoms occurring during exercise (25). The origin and course of the coronary arteries should then be investigated by selective echocardiographic study of the aortic root and eventually by coronary angiography. Disqualification from sports is the simplest preventive measure. Surgery is now feasible with different techniques including aorta-coronary bypass, reimplantation of the anomalous vessel and osteoplasty (26).

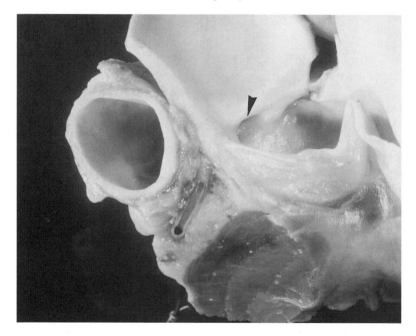

Figure 3. Sudden arrhythmic death due to anomalous origin of the left coronary artery from the right sinus in an 1-year-old soccer player. View of the aortic root: the left coronary ostium is located in the right sinus of Valsalva (arrow). Note the course of the left main trunk between the aorta and the pulmonary artery.

The intramyocardial course of the coronary artery is still a controversial cause of sudden death, even though recent clinical studies have unequivocally demonstrated that a myocardial bridge can lead to myocardial ischemia (8, 14, 27, 28). The role of intramyocardial course in precipitating sudden death during strenuous exercise was confirmed pathologically by Morales *et al.* (28), who found ischemic injury at various stages in the myocardium supplied by the intramural coronary artery. Persistent diastolic impairment of the coronary segment is the most reasonable explanation of myocardial ischemia, taking into account that coronary blood perfusion occurs mostly during diastole (29). In our experience of sudden death in the young, the intramural course was long and deep and the affected vessel was usually the left anterior descending coronary artery (14, 68) (Fig. 4). We recently observed a distinctive histologic feature consisting of a myocardial sheath encircling the intramural coronary segment with myocardial disarray and interstitial fibrosis, which may act as a restrictive perivascular ring impairing diastolic blood flow, especially during physical exercise when there is an increased heart rate and myocardial oxygen request. Surgical debridging or intracoronary stenting may be advisable in patients who are at risk.

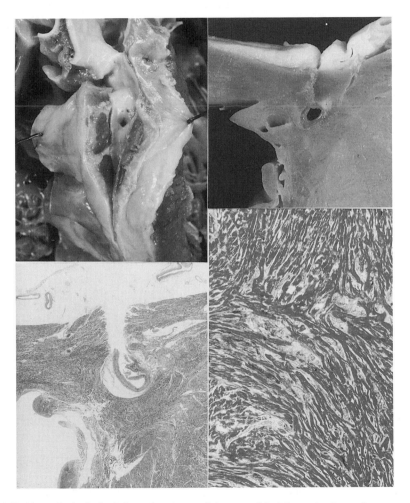

Figure 4. Sudden arrhythmic death due to intramyocardial course of the left anterior descending coronary artery in a 35-year-old runner. (A) Opened left anterior descending coronary artery: note the long and deep intramyocardial course. (B) Cross section of the same showing a thick myocardial bridge. (C) Corresponding histology in panoramic view (Heidenhain trichrome, o.m. original x 9). (D) Close-up of the myocardium surrounding the intramural coronary segment showing fibrosis and disarray (Heidenhain trichrome, o.m. original x 45).

Arrhythmogenic Right Ventricular Cardiomyopathy

Arrhythmogenic right ventricular cardiomyopathy is a primary heart muscle disorder, recently discovered and introduced in the World Health Organization's classification of cardiomyopathies. It is often associated with autosomal inheritance (30, 31). It is characterized by a fibro-fatty progressive atrophy of the right ventricular myocardium, accounting for ominous arrhythmias that put the individual at risk of cardiac arrest (12, 32, 33) (Figs. 5-7). Various genes have been mapped in different chromosomes, but so far none has been identified (34-39). Since the left ventricle is usually spared, unaware affected subjects may undertake even strenuous exercise. On macroscopic examination, massive regional or diffuse fibro-fatty replacement, parchment-like and translucent appearance of the right ventricular free wall and mild to moderate ventricular dilatation together with inferior, apical or infundibular aneurysms, are often observed (32) (Fig. 6).

Histologically fibro-fatty infiltration is usually associated with focal myocardial degeneration and necrosis and patchy inflammatory infiltrates (32) (Fig. 7). Progressive myocyte loss has recently been ascribed to apoptosis (programmed cell death), probably triggered by T-lymphocyte infiltrates (40, 41). Viral infection and humoral autoimmunity as possible causes have been ruled out so far (30).

The high electrical vulnerability in these patients is easily explained by the widespread, irregular disruption of the right ventricular myocardium, accounting for inhomogeneous electrical conduction and activation, which predisposes the patients to the onset of malignant reentrant ventricular tachyarrhythmias (42).

As previously stated, the occurrence of sudden death due to arrhythmogenic right ventricular cardiomyopathy is significantly increased in athletes (43, 44). Risk factors for sudden death include young age, malignant family history, previous cardiac arrest, syncope, ventricular tachyarrhythmias, extensive myocardial involvement, QT dispersion ⩾80 msec and strenuous exercise. The propensity for arrhythmogenic right ventricular cardiomyopathy to precipitate arrhythmic cardiac arrest during physical exercise is most likely linked to both hemodynamic and neurohumoral factors. Physical exercise results

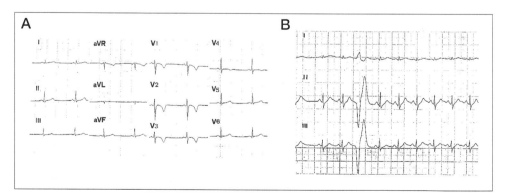

Figure 5. Sudden arrhythmic death due to arrhythmogenic right ventricular cardiomyopathy in a 17-year-old soccer player. (A) 12-lead basal electrocardiogram showing inverted T-waves in right precordial leads in V1-V4. (B) Isolated premature ventricular beat recorded on peripheral leads during exercise electrocardiogram.

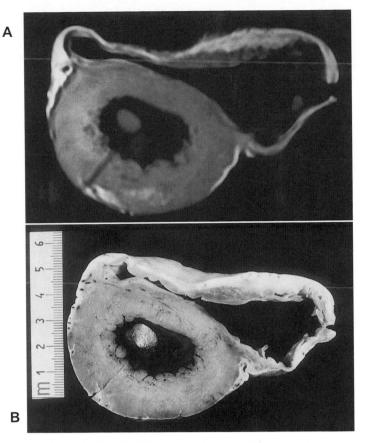

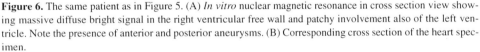

Figure 6. The same patient as in Figure 5. (A) *In vitro* nuclear magnetic resonance in cross section view showing massive diffuse bright signal in the right ventricular free wall and patchy involvement also of the left ventricle. Note the presence of anterior and posterior aneurysms. (B) Corresponding cross section of the heart specimen.

in an acute, disproportionate increase in right ventricular afterload and cavity enlargement, which may trigger ventricular arrhythmias by stretching the residual right ventricular myocytes (45-47). Progression of the disease from the epicardium to the endocardium might account for a functional and/or structural sympathetic denervation with supersensitivity to catecholamines and enhanced arrhythmogenicity during sympathetic stimulation (48, 49).

The early identification of arrhythmogenic right ventricular cardiomyopathy is a challenge. Most athletes who die suddenly from arrhythmogenic right ventricular cardiomyopathy had a history of signs and symptoms of ventricular electrical instability, such as palpitations, overlooked syncopal episodes and ventricular arrhythmias with left bundle branch block morphology. Moreover, distinctive findings at the basal ECG were present in 50% of the cases, consisting of inverted T-waves in right precordial leads (17) (Fig. 5). A family history of juvenile sudden death is strongly suspicious (50). Despite an apparently normal heart size on chest x-ray, echocardiography may show regional or global

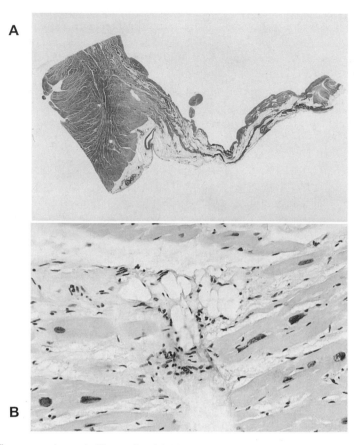

Figure 7. The same patient as in Figures 5 and 6. (A) Panoramic histological section of the posterior wall of the right ventricle disclosing fibrofatty replacement and aneurysms (Heidenhain trichrome, o.m. original x 3). (B) At higher magnification, inflammatory infiltrates with adipocytes and fibrous tissue replacing the myocytes (hematoxylin-eosin, o.m. original x 240).

right ventricular enlargement, as well as structural abnormalities in wall motion (51). Magnetic resonance imaging may help to detect fatty tissue infiltration (52) and, in selected cases, right ventricular angiography (53) and endomyocardial biopsy (54) may be indicated for final diagnosis. Diagnostic criteria have been proposed for the *in vivo* detection of the disease (55).

Hypertrophic Cardiomyopathy

Hypertrophic cardiomyopathy is usually an inherited heart muscle disease, characterized by a concentric hypertrophy of the left ventricle. Several missense mutations of genes encoding for proteins of cardiac sarcomere, such as beta-myosin heavy chain, cardiac troponin T, alfa-tropomyosin and myosin-binding protein C have been identified in the familiar forms (56). Hypertrophic cardiomyopathy has been suggested as the principal cause of sudden death of athletes in the United States, with a prevalence of up to 50% of sports-related cardiac fatalities (3). Gross pathologic features include increased heart weight, left ventricular hypertrophy with asymmetric septal thickness (Fig. 8) and frequently a subaortic plaque associated with a thickening of the anterior leaflet of the mitral valve, as a result of systolic anterior motion and dynamic left ventricular outflow tract obstruction (3, 6, 10, 57, 58).

The histological hallmark of the disease is the bizarre and disordered arrangement of myocytes (myocardial disarray) associated with diffuse interstitial and replacement-type fibrosis (57) (Fig. 8). The small intramural coronary arteries often show a dysplastic tunica media with intimal proliferation, which in our experience, however, rarely reaches obstructive degree. In young subjects who died suddenly, histological signs of acute (contraction band and coagulation necrosis) and/or healed (extensive replacement fibrosis) ischemic injury were observed, mostly within the septal hypertrophy (68).

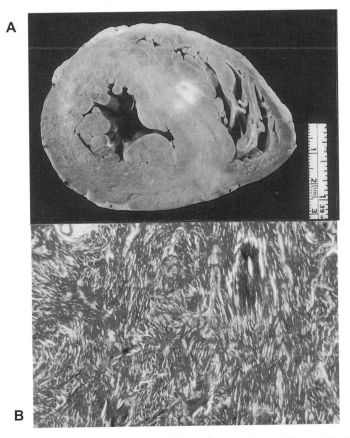

Figure 8. Sudden arrhythmic death due to hypertrophic cardiomyopathy in a 19-year-old soldier during gymnastics. (A) Cross section showing asymmetric septal hypertrophy centered by a large scar. (B) Histology of the ventricular septum shows myocardial disarray and extensive replacement-type fibrosis (Heidenhain trichrome, o.m. original x 180).

Myocardial ischemia has been related to small vessel disease (59) but in our opinion its observation in the hypertrophied and disarranged septal myocardium suggests that increased myocardial stiffness and intramural diastolic pressure may critically impair diastolic compliance and capillary blood filling.

Risk factors for sudden death in hypertrophic cardiomyopathy include young age, malignant family history, adverse genotype, previous cardiac arrest or sustained ventricular tachycardia (VT), recurrent syncope, nonsustained VT on Holter monitoring, massive left ventricular hypertrophy (>35 mm), myocardial ischemia and exercise performance (56).

Left ventricular hypertrophy, in the absence of systemic hypertension and histologic evidence of disarray, has occasionally been seen in athletes who died suddenly and has been labeled as idiopathic left ventricular hypertrophy (3). The degree of hypertrophy is well beyond that seen in physiologic hypertrophy of the athlete's heart. Unlike hypertrophic cardiomyopathy, the hypertrophy is concentric and symmetrical and there is no evidence of genetic transmission. This condition may represent a nonfamilial variant of hypertrophic cardiomyopathy.

The mechanism of sudden death in athletes with hypertrophic cardiomyopathy has been ascribed to primary ventricular arrhythmias, the substrate consisting of dysplastic myocardium with a disarray feature. Other postulated mechanisms include paroxysmal supraventricular arrhythmias (atrial fibrillation) (60), atrioventricular block and hypotension caused by an inappropriate vasodilator response to exercise (61). The observation of ischemic myocardial damage, either acute or chronic, supports the hypothesis that myocardial ischemia plays an important role in the progressive loss of myocardium and in the onset of life-threatening ventricular arrhythmias (62).

In the Veneto region study, hypertrophic cardiomyopathy caused only one death among 49 athletes (17). One may wonder whether this reflects a lower prevalence of the disease in our country. In the USA, hypertrophic cardiomyopathy is present in approximately 0.2% of young adults who are screened by echocardiography and the prevalence is higher among blacks (0.25%) than among whites (0.10%) (63). A prevalence of 0.07% was found among the white athletes screened mostly by electrocardiography in the Veneto region, a figure quite similar to that reported among young white persons in the USA. Moreover, hypertrophic cardiomyopathy caused sudden death in the nonathletic young population with a prevalence similar to that found in the USA. Indeed, the prevalence of hypertrophic cardiomyopathy among young nonathletes was similar in our study (7.3%) and in the study of Burke *et al.* in the USA (3%), whereas it was quite different among young athletes who died suddenly (2% *vs.* 24%, respectively) (8, 17). Since competitive athletes undergo systematic preparticipation screening in Italy, it is likely that a selective reduction in sudden death for hypertrophic cardiomyopathy is ascribable to identification and disqualification of affected athletes.

Other Cardiovascular Diseases

MITRAL VALVE PROLAPSE

Mitral valve prolapse is a minor cause of sudden death in athletes, despite its high prevalence in the general population (6, 7, 17). In our experience, it accounted for 10% of all fatalities among the athlete subgroup. The mechanism is clearly arrhythmic and many possible explanations have been advanced, such as endocardial valve friction and coronary microembolism from platelet valve deposits, as well as concealed disease, such as conduction system abnormalities, hypertrophic and arrhythmogenic right ventricular cardiomyopathies (64, 65). Significant fatty dystrophy of the right ventricular free wall has recently been reported in 70% of sudden death victims with mitral valve prolapse, indicating the right ventricle as a possible source of life-threatening ventricular arrhythmias (Fig. 9). Whether this fatty infiltration may be related or not to arrhythmogenic right ventricular cardiomyopathy remains to be elucidated.

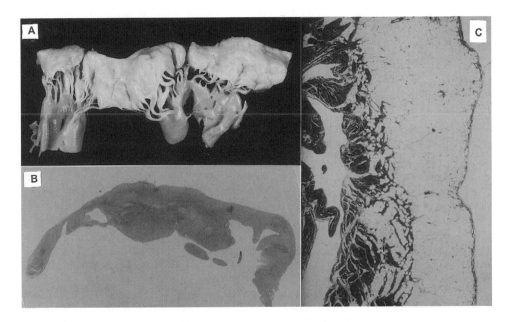

Figure 9. Sudden arrhythmic death due to mitral valve prolapse in a 23-year-old tennis player with Marfan's syndrome. (A) Excised prolapsing mitral valve: note thickened and mucoid valve leaflets. (B) Histology showing extensive myxoid degeneration of the fibrosa (Alcian-periodic acid-Schiff, o.m. original x 18). (C) Fibrofatty replacement of the right ventricular free wall (Heidenhain trichrome, o.m. original x 180).

CONDUCTION SYSTEM ABNORMALITIES

Apart from overt preexcitation syndromes, such as Wolff-Parkinson-White syndrome or Low-Ganong-Levine syndrome, with a definitive ECG pattern of short P-R interval, with or without delta wave respectively, we reported three cases with apparently normal hearts at both gross and routine histologic examination and conduction system abnormalities at histologic serial sections study, consisting of septal (atrioventricular and nodoventricular) accessory pathways in two and sclerocalcific interruption of His's bundle and branches in one. The significance of these occult conduction system abnormalities (or possibly normal variants) as well as the possibility of an *in vivo* identification remain intriguing in the absence of prodromal symptoms and ECG recordings.

MYOCARDITIS

In our experience, myocarditis was a not so negligible cause of sudden death, either in athletes or in nonathletes (6, 66). It accounted for 6.1% and 8.2% of all fatalities respectively, clearly indicating an independence from exercise (17). Death is usually instantaneous in poorly symptomatic patients or in those with a flue-like syndrome, suggesting an abrupt ventricular fibrillation. The heart was grossly normal in most of the cases and at histology foci of lymphocytic or polymorphous inflammatory infiltrates with myocardial necrosis were visible (67) (Fig. 10). Massive infiltrates, similar to those seen in fulminant myocarditis with cardiogenic shock, were exceptionally observed. Concomitant areas of replacement type fibrosis suggest a subacute chronic form. The inflammation, either in its active or healed patterns, may provide a concealed substrate for the onset of ominous ventricular arrhythmias. Fatal events in athletes due to myocarditis seem unpredictable, since this disease is mostly silent. Viral infections of the myocardium are the most plausible cause. Molecular biology techniques with polymerase chain reaction are now essential tools and the gold-standard for an etiological diagnosis.

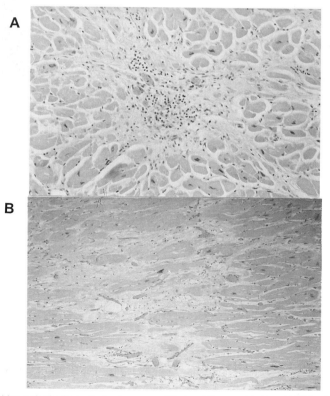

Figure 10. Sudden arrhythmic death due to myocarditis in a 24-year-old skier. (A) Histology of the ventricular myocardium showing patchy nodular lymphocytic infiltrates (hematoxylin-eosin, o.m. original x 150). (B) Replacement-type fibrosis and myocyte hypertrophy: the histologic finding are in keeping with chronic myocarditis (hematoxylin-eosin, o.m. original x 75).

AORTIC DISSECTION

Aortic dissection occurred as a consequence of spontaneous laceration of the ascending aorta in a Marfan soccer player, with rupture into the pericardial cavity, cardiac tamponade and electromechanical dissociation (Fig. 11).

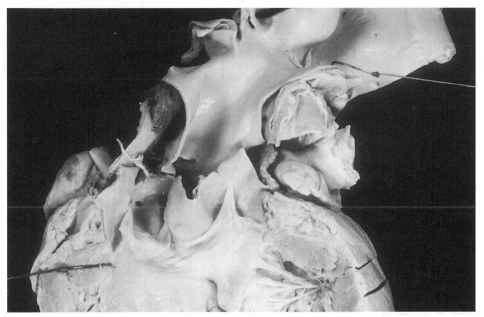

Figure 11. Sudden mechanical death due to aortic dissection in a 28-year-old player with Marfan's syndrome. Note the spontaneous laceration of the ascending aorta with aortic rupture and cardiac tamponade.

The basic defect consisted of elastic fragmentation and atrophy of the tunica media with medionecrosis leading to aortic wall fragility. The disease is rarely isolated in the young and is usually associated with congenital cardiovascular defects such as Marfan's syndrome, aortic coarctation and/or bicuspid aortic valve (68-79). Highly static, isometric sports performance, with a sudden increase of systemic blood pressure, may favor the rupture.

Cross-sectional echocardiography of the aortic root may be of help in detecting dilatation and in indirectly indicating the risk of rupture. Of course, tissue characterization of the aortic wall should be the gold standard and a high frequency ultrasonic technique has been recently advanced as a promising tool for the *in vivo* identification of elastic atrophy in the aortic tunica media (74).

Pathology of Sudden Death in Athletes: USA *vs*. European Perspectives

There are no epidemiologic data to confirm that sudden death in athletes occurs more frequently in the USA than in Italy and this is related to the rigorous preparticipation screening which is carried out in Italy, theoretically much more able to identify and disqualify athletes at risk. Nonetheless, although sudden death in young competitive athletes was mostly cardiovascular and related to the same spectrum of disease on both sides of the ocean, the prevalence of the various causes differs substantially.

Whereas sudden death due to arrhythmogenic right ventricular cardiomyopathy was anecdotal in the US series (3, 6, 10, 11), in our experience it was the third cause of sudden death among the nonathletes and the first cause among the athletes, disclosing a clear-cut association with effort (17). Notably, athletes who died due to arrhythmogenic right ventricular cardiomyopathy, although having presented a history of syncopal episodes, ECG abnormalities consisting of inverted T-waves in the right precordial leads and ventricular arrhythmias with a left bundle-branch block morphology, were not identified at preparticipation screening because signs and symptoms were overlooked due to the scarce awareness of the disease and the absence of diagnostic criteria. The results of our study suggest that the finding at ECG of even isolated premature ventricular beat with morphologic features of left bundle branch block associated with right precordial T-wave abnormalities, with or without a history of syncopal attacks, should suggest at cardiovascular screening the possibility of an underlying arrhythmogenic right ventricular cardiomyopathy and lead to additional testing such as echocardiography.

The high incidence of arrhythmogenic right ventricular cardiomyopathy in the Italian series may be due to genetic factors. The disease is endemic in our region, with a prevalence of 6 per 10,000 (41). However, the concept of arrhythmogenic right ventricular cardiomyopathy as a peculiarly Venetian disease is misleading, since there is growing evidence that the disease is worldwide yet still largely under-diagnosed at both clinical and postmortem investigation (75). Consequently, comparison of the results of our investigation with those of previous studies on sudden death in athletes in the USA, is limited by the fact that arrhythmogenic right ventricular cardiomyopathy is a condition that has only recently been discovered. The accuracy of autopsy and the interpretation of pathologic findings may also play a crucial role in establishing the causes of sudden death. Arrhythmogenic right ventricular cardiomyopathy is rarely associated with cardiomegaly and usually spares the coronary arteries and the left ventricle so that hearts may be erroneously considered normal. In the Veneto region, the accuracy of postmortem studies is ensured by the awareness and knowledge of the disease, whereas forensic pathologists elsewhere, by searching for the cause of death in the left systemic ventricle, may fail to pay attention to focal or diffuse fibro-fatty dystrophy of the right pulmonary ventricle. Finally, the disease is still poorly identified in the clinical setting and subtle signs and symptoms are often overlooked; thus sports qualification is still granted (17). It is likely that in the past, a number of sudden deaths in young competitive athletes in the USA may have been due to an under-recognized arrhythmogenic right ventricular cardiomyopathy.

The second striking feature is the low prevalence of hypertrophic cardiomyopathy in the series of young competitive athletes who died suddenly in the Veneto region (17). Again, racial factors may have influenced the results. The population of the Veneto region is homogeneously white. In the USA, blacks who died during exercise had a greater incidence of hypertrophic cardiomyopathy than whites. However, a similar prevalence of hypertrophic cardiomyopathy as a cause of nonsports-related sudden death in the nonathletic young population in the USA and Italy (8, 17) suggests a selective reduction of sudden death from hypertrophic cardiomyopathy in competitive athletes who undergo the systematic preparticipation screening that has been taking place for more than 20 years in our country. The protocol for cardiovascular preparticipation screening for competitive athletes in Italy includes, on an annual basis and as a rule, family and personal clinical history, physical examination including blood pressure, basal 12-lead ECG, limited exercise testing ECG and additional investigations if indicated (echocardiogram, Holter monitoring, maximal exercise testing) (76, 77). Hypertrophic cardiomyopathy is suspected at the initial screening of young people with a suggestive personal or family history and positive physical or ECG findings. Basal ECG has been reported to be very sensitive and it is abnormal in approximately 95% of patients with hypertrophic cardiomyopathy, leading to further noninvasive study such as echocardiography with easy detection of asymmetric left ventricular hypertrophy (17). The definitive diagnosis is subsequently achieved by echocardiographic demonstration of a hypertrophic, nondilated left ventricle, in the absence of other cardiac or systemic diseases that could cause hypertrophy. In our study, of the 33,735 athletes initially screened, 3,016 (8.9%) were referred for echocardiography and 22 were eventually found to have evidence of hypertrophic cardiomyopathy and were disqualified (17). Was this effective in preventing sudden death for hypertrophic cardiomyopathy? None of the disqualified athletes with hypertrophic cardiomyopathy died during a mean follow-up period of 8.2 ± 5 years. Thus, according to our findings, identification and disqualification of athletes found to be affected by hypertrophic cardiomyopathy at preparticipation screening seems to prevent sudden death.

Why is hypertrophic cardiomyopathy still so frequent as a cause of sudden deaths in US athletes? Cardiovascular preparticipation screening of competitive athletes in the USA is such that most athletes with hypertrophic cardiomyopathy may escape identification (78, 79). Neither basal ECG nor echocardiography are regularly carried out during screening. According to the American Heart Association, based on both practical and cost-effectiveness considerations, routine use of 12-lead ECG, echocardiography and exercise testing ECG are not recommended at population screening (78). Medical history and physical examination is considered to be the most practical and available approach to the screening of competitive sports participants. It may even be acceptable for an appropriately trained registered nurse or physician's assistant to perform screening examinations. No laboratory investigations are planned.

Screening is clearly a matter of costs. In Italy most of the expense of screening competitive athletes is covered by the National Health Service, individuals making only a small contribution ($40 for obligatory and $40 for additional investigations in subjects older than 18 years, $4 for each in subjects younger than 18). In the USA the entire cost of any examination must be covered by the individual, thus rendering laboratory investigations noncompulsory. It was quite rewarding to realize that our systematic preparticipation screening was so effective, not only in identifying and disqualifying the athletes affected by hypertrophic cardiomyopathy but also in preventing sudden death, since none of the disqualified athletes with hypertrophic cardiomyopathy died during a mean follow-up period of eight years.

Conclusions

Monitoring of sudden death in young people of the Veneto region in Italy, a well-defined geographic area populated by a homogeneous ethnic group, where a systematic preparticipation athletic screening has been a practice for 20 years, has demonstrated that the prevalence of cardiovascular causes of sudden death in young competitive athletes differs from that previously reported in the USA (17). Hypertrophic cardiomyopathy has been a very uncommon cause of fatal events, most likely due to the identification and disqualification of affected subjects, who are still alive after a mean follow-up of 8 years.

These findings are strongly in favor of the effectiveness of the Italian protocol for preparticipation screening in preventing sudden death in young athletes affected by hypertrophic cardiomyopathy.

Arrhythmogenic right ventricular cardiomyopathy, a still poorly recognized clinico-pathologic entity, was the most frequent cardiovascular disease leading to sports-related cardiac arrest. Unlike coronary artery disease, both atherosclerotic and congenital, fatal arrhythmogenic right ventricular cardiomyopathy may have been suspected at preparticipation athletic screening on the basis of arrhythmic prodromal symptoms and ECG signs. With increased awareness of the diagnostic criteria for arrhythmogenic right ventricular cardiomyopathy, more athletes at risk will be identified in the future and sudden death possibly prevented.

Acknowledgements

This work was supported by grants from the Veneto region, the Research Project on Juvenile Sudden Death, Venice, Italy, the National Research Council and the MURST Project on Myocardial Infarction, Rome, Italy.

References

1. Buddington, R.S., Stahl, C.J.I., McAllister, H.A. *Sports, death and unusual heart disease*. Am J Cardiol 1974, 33: 129.
2. Thompson, P.D., Stern, M.P., Williams, P., Duncan, K., Haskell, W.L., Wood, P.D. *Death during jogging or running: A study of 18 cases*. JAMA 1979, 242: 1265.
3. Maron, B.J., Roberts, W.C., McAllister, H.A., Rosing, D.R., Epstein, S.E. *Sudden death in young athletes*. Circulation 1980, 62: 218-29.
4. Waller, B.F., Roberts, W.C. *Sudden death while running in conditioned runners aged 40 years or over*. Am J Cardiol 1980, 45: 1292.
5. Virmani, R., Robinowitz, M., McAllister, H.A. *Nontraumatic death in joggers*. Am J Med 1982, 72: 874.
6. Maron, B.J., Epstein, S.E., Roberts, W.C. *Causes of sudden death in competitive athletes*. J Am Coll Cardiol 1986, 7: 204.
7. Corrado, D., Thiene, G., Nava, A., Pennelli, N., Rossi L. *Sudden death in young competitive athletes: Clinico-pathologic correlations in 22 cases*. Am J Med 1990, 89: 588-96.
8. Burke, A.P., Farb, A., Virmani, R., Goodin, J., Smialek, J.E. *Sports-related and non-sports-related sudden cardiac death in young adults*. Am Heart J 1991, 121: 568.
9. Van Camp, S.P., Bloor, C.M., Mueller, F.O., Cantu, R.C., Olson, H.G., *Non-traumatic sports death in high school and college athletes*. Med Sci Sports Exerc, 1995, 27: 641-7.

10. Maron, B.J., Shirani, J., Poliac, L.C., Mathenge, R., Roberts, W.C., Mueller, F.O. *Sudden death in young competitive athletes. Clinical, demographic, and pathological profiles.* JAMA 1996, 276: 199-204.
11. Maron, B.J., Roberts, W.C., Epstein, S.E. *Sudden death in hypertrophic cardiomyopathy: A profile of 78 patients.* Circulation 1982, 65: 1388.
12. Thiene, G., Nava, A., Corrado, D., Rossi, L., Pennelli, N. *Right ventricular cardiomyopathy and sudden death in young people.* N Engl J Med 1988, 318: 129-33.
13. Virmani, R., Rogan, K., Cheitlin, M.D. *Congenital coronary artery anomalies: Pathologic aspects.* In: Nonatherosclerotic Ischemic Heart Disease R. Virmani, M.B. Forman (Eds.). Raven Press: New York 1989: 153.
14. Corrado, D., Thiene, G., Cocco, P., Frescura, C. *Non-atherosclerotic coronary artery disease and sudden death in the young.* Br Heart J 1992, 68: 601-7.
15. Topaz, O., Edwards, J.E. *Pathologic features of sudden death in children, adolescents, and young adults.* Chest 1985, 87: 476-82.
16. Thiene, G., Pennelli, N., Rossi, L. *Cardiac conduction system abnormalities as a possible cause of sudden death in young athletes.* Hum Pathol 1983, 14: 70-4.
17. Corrado, D., Basso, C., Schiavon, M., Thiene, G. *Screening for hypertrophic cardiomyopathy in young athletes.* N Engl J Med 1998, 339: 364-9.
18. Noakes, T.D., Opie, H.L., Rose, A.G., Kleynhans, P.H., Schepers, N.J., Dowdeswell R. *Autopsy-proved coronary atherosclerosis in marathon runners.* N Engl J Med 1979, 310: 86-9.
19. Ciampricotti, R., El Gamal, M., Relik, T., et al. *Clinical characteristics and coronary angiographic findings of patients with unstable angina, acute myocardial infarction, and survivors of sudden ischemic death occurring during or after sport.* Am Heart J 1990, 120: 1267-78.
20. Corrado, D., Thiene, G., Pennelli, N. *Sudden death as the first manifestation of coronary artery disease in young people (<35 years).* Eur Heart J 1988, 9: 139-44.
21. Corrado, D., Basso, C., Poletti, A., Angelini, A., Valente, M., Thiene, G. *Sudden death in the young. Is coronary thrombosis the major precipitating factor?* Circulation 1994, 90: 2315-23.
22. Cheitlin, M.D., De Castro, C.M., McAllister, H.A. *Sudden death as a complication of anomalous left coronary origin from the anterior sinus of Valsalva: A not so minor congenital anomaly.* Circulation 1994, 50: 780-7.
23. Roberts, W.C., Siegel, R.J., Zipes, D.P. *Origin of the right coronary artery from the left sinus of Valsalva and its functional consequences: Analysis of 10 necropsy patients.* Am J Cardiol 1982, 49: 863-8
24. Frescura, C., Basso, C., Thiene, G. *Anomalous origin of coronary arteries and risk of sudden death: A study based on an autopsy population of congenital heart disease.* Hum Pathol 1998, 29: 689-95.
25. Basso, C., Maron, B.J., Corrado, D., Thiene, G. *Clinical profile of congenital coronary artery anomalies with origin from the wrong aortic sinus leading to sudden death in young competitive athletes.* Circulation 1998, 98: 1-618.
26. Cohen, A.J., Grishkin, B.A., Hestel, R.A., Head, H.D. *Surgical therapy in the management of coronary anomalies.* Ann Thorac Surg 1989, 47: 630-7.
27. Vasan, R.S., Bahl, V.K., Rajani, M. *Myocardial infarction associated with a myocardial bridge.* Int J Cardiol 1989, 25: 240-1.
28. Morales, A.R., Romanelli, R., Boucek, R.J. *The mural left anterior descending coronary artery, strenous exercise and sudden death.* Circulation 1980, 62: 250-7.
29. Ge, J., Erbel, R., Rupprecht, H.J., et al. *Comparison of intravascular ultrasound and angiography in the assessment of myocardial bridging.* Circulation 1994, 89: 1725-32.
30. Nava, A., Rossi, L., Thiene, G. (Eds). Arrhythmogenic Right Ventricular Cardiomyopathy/dysplasia. Elsevier: Amsterdam 1997.
31. Richardson, P., McKenna, W.J., Bristow, et al. *Report of the 1995 WHO/ISFC Task Force on the definition and classification of cardiomyopathies.* Circulation 1996, 93: 841-2.
32. Basso, C., Thiene, G., Corrado, D., Angelini, A., Nava, A., Valente, M. *Arrhythmogenic right ventricular cardiomyopathy: Dysplasia, dystrophy, or myocarditis?* Circulation 1996, 94: 983-91.
33. Marcus, F.I., Fontaine, G.H., Guiraudon, G., et al. *Right ventricular dysplasia: A report of 24 cases.* Circulation 1982, 65: 384-98.
34. Rampazzo, A., Nava, A., Danieli, G.A., et al. *The gene for arrhythmogenic right ventricular cardiomyopathy maps to chromosome 14q23-q24.* Hum Mol Genet 1994, 3: 959-62.
35. Rampazzo, A., Nava, A., Erne, P., et al. *A new locus for arrhythmogenic right ventricular cardiomyopathy (ARVD2) maps to chromosome 1q42-q43.* Hum Mol Genet 1995, 4: 2151-4.

36. Severini, G.M., Kraijinovic, M., Pinamonti, B., et al. *A new locus for arrhythmogenic right ventricular dysplasia on the long arm of chromosome 14*. Genomics 1996, 31: 193-200.

37. Rampazzo, A., Nava, A., Miorin, M., et al. *ARVD4, a new locus for arrhythmogenic right ventricular cardiomyopathy, maps to chromosome 2 long arm*. Genomics 1997, 45: 259-63.

38. Coonar, A.S., Protonotarios, N., Tsatsopoulou, A., et al. *Gene for arrhythmogenic right ventricular cardiomyopathy with diffuse nonepidermolytic palmoplantar keratoderma and woolly hair (Naxos disease) maps to 17q21*. Circulation 1998, 97: 2049-58.

39. Ahmad, F., Duanxiang, Li., Karibe, A., et al. *Localization of a gene responsible for arrhythmogenic right ventricular dysplasia to chromosome 3p23*. Circulation 1998, 98: 2705-91.

40. Mallat, Z., Tedgui, A., Fontaliran, F., Frank, R., Durigon, M., Fontaine, G. *Evidence of apoptosis in arrhythmogenic right ventricular dysplasia*. N Engl J Med 1996, 335: 1190-6.

41. Valente, M., Calabrese, F., Thiene, G., et al. In vivo *evidence of apoptosis in arrhythmogenic right ventricular cardiomyopathy*. Am J Pathol 1998, 152: 479-84.

42. Fontaine, G., Frank, R., Tonet, J.L., et al. *Arrhythmogenic right ventricular dysplasia; a clinical model for the study of chronic ventricular tachycardia*. Jpn J Circ 1984, 48: 515-38.

43. Furlanello, F., Bettini, R., Cozzi, F., et al. *Ventricular arrhythmias and sudden death in athletes*. Ann NY Acad Sci 1984, 427: 253-62.

44. Furlanello, F., Bertoldi, A., Bettini, R., Durante, G.B., Vergara, G. *The disease in competitive athletes*. In: Arrhythmogenic Right Ventricular Cardiomyopathy/Dysplasia. A. Nava, L. Rossi, G. Thiene (Eds.). Elsevier: Amsterdam 1997, 477-87.

45. Douglas, P.S., O'Toole, M.L., Hiller, W.D.B., Reichek N. *Different effects of prolonged exercise on the right and left ventricles*. J Am Coll Cardiol 1990, 15: 64-9.

46. Gurtner, H.P., Walser, P., Fassler, B. *Normal values for pulmonary hemodynamics at rest and during exercise in man*. Prog Respir Res 1975, 9: 295-315.

47. Stanek, V., Widirnsky, J., Degre, S., Denolin, H. *The lesser circulation during exercise in healthy subjects*. Prog Respir Res 1975, 9: 1-9.

48. Inoue, H., Zipes, D.P. *Results of sympathetic denervation in the canine heart: Supersensitivity that may be arrhythmogenic*. Circulation 1987, 75: 877-87.

49. Wichter, T., Hindricks, G., Lerch, H., et al. *Regional myocardial sympathetic dysinnervation in arrhythmogenic right ventricular cardiomyopathy*. Circulation 1994, 89: 667-83.

50. Nava, A., Thiene, G., Canciani, B., et al. *Familial occurrence of right ventricular dysplasia: A study of nine families*. J Am Coll Cardiol 1988, 12: 1222-8.

51. Blomstrom-Lundqvist, C., Selin, K., Jonsson, R., Johansson, S.R., Schlossman, D., Olsson S.B. *Cardioangiographic findings in patients with arrhythmogenic right ventricular dysplasia*. Br Heart J 1988, 59: 556-63.

52. Menghetti, L., Basso, C., Nava, A., Angelini, A., Thiene, G. *Spin-echo nuclear magnetic resonance for tissue characterization in arrhythmogenic right ventricular cardiomyopathy*. Heart 1997, 76: 467-70.

53. Daliento, L., Rizzoli, G., Thiene, G., et al. *Diagnostic accuracy of right ventricular ventriculography in arrhythmogenic right ventricular cardiomyopathy*. Am J Cardiol 1990, 66: 741-5.

54. Angelini, A., Basso, C., Nava, A., Thiene, G. *Endomyocardial biopsy in arrhythmogenic right ventricular cardiomyopathy*. Am Heart J 1996, 132: 203-6.

55. McKenna, W.J., Thiene, G,. Nava, A., et al. *Diagnosis of arrhythmogenic right ventricular dysplasia/ cardiomyopathy*. Br Heart J 1994, 71: 215-8.

56. Spirito, P., Seidnma, C.E., McKenna, W.J., Maron, B.J. *The management of hypertrophic cardiomyopathy*. N Engl J Med 1997, 336: 775-85.

57. Maron, B.J., Roberts, W.C. *Quantitative analysis of cardiac muscle cell disorganization in the ventricular septum of patients with hypertrophic cardiomyopathy*. Circulation 1979, 59: 689.

58. Davies, M.J. McKenna, W.J. *Hypertrophic cardiomyopathy-pathology and pathogenesis*. Histopathology 1995, 26: 493-500.

59. Maron, B.J., Wolfson, J.K., Epstein, S.E., Roberts, W.C. *Intramural ("small vessel") coronary artery disease in hypertrophic cardiomyopathy*. J Am Coll Cardiol 1986, 8: 545-57.

60. Krikler, D.M., Davies, M.J., Rowland, W., Goodwin, J.F., Evans, R.C., Shaw, D.B. *Sudden death in hypertrophic cardiomyopathy associated accessory atrioventricular pathways*. Br Heart J 1980, 43: 245-51.

61. Frenneaux, M.P., Counihan, P.J., Caforio, A.L.P., Chikamori, T., McKenna, W.J. *Abnormal blood pressure response during exercise in hypertrophic cardiomyopathy* Circulation 1990, 82: 1995-2002.

62. Basso, C., Corrado, D., Nava, A., Thiene, G. *Hypertrophic cardiomyopathy: Pathologic evidence of myocardial ischemic injury in young sudden death victims.* Circulation 1996, 94: 1-427

63. Maron, B.J., Gardin, J.M., Flack, J.M., Gidding, S.S., Kurosaki, T.T., Bild, D.E. *Prevalence of hypertrophic cardiomyopathy in a general population of young adults: Echocardiographic analysis of 4111 subjects in CARDIA study.* Circulation 1995, 92: 785-9

64. Corrado, D., Basso, C., Nava, A., Rossi, L., Thiene, G. *Sudden death in young people with apparently isolated mitral valve prolapse.* G Ital Cardiol 1997, 27: 1097-105.

65. Martini, B., Basso, C., Thiene, G. *Sudden death in mitral valve prolapse with Holter monitoring-documented ventricular fibrillation evidence of coexisting arrhythmogenic right ventricular cardiomyopathy.* Int J Cardiol 1995, 49: 274-8.

66. Frustaci, A., Bellocci, F., Olsen, E.G.J. *Results of biventricular endomyocardial biopsy in survivors of cardiac arrest with apparently normal hearts.* Am J Cardiol 1994, 74: 890-5.

67. Corrado, D., Basso, C., Thiene, G. *Sudden cardiac death in young people with normal heart. Is the heart truly normal?* Circulation 1998, 98: 1-93.

68. Basso, C., Frescura, C., Corrado, et al. *Congenital heart disease and sudden death in the young.* Hum Pathol 1995, 26: 1065-72.

69. Pachulski, R.T., Weinberg, A.L., Chan, K.W. *Aortic aneurysm in patients with functionally normal or minimally stenotic bicuspid aortic valve.* Am J Cardiol 1991, 67: 781-2.

70. Edwards, J.E. *Aneurysms of the thoracic aorta complicating coarctation.* Circulation 1972, 48: 195-201.

71. Edwards, W.D., Leaf, D.S., Edwards, J.E. *Dissecting aortic aneurysm associated with congenital bicuspid aortic valve.* Circulation 1978, 57: 1022-5.

72. Roberts, C.S., Roberts, W.C. *Dissection of the aorta associated with congenital malformation of aortic valve.* J Am Coll Cardiol 1991, 17: 712-6.

73. Roberts, W.C., Honig, H.S. *The spectrum of cardiovascular disease in the Marfan syndrome: A clinicopathologic study of 18 necropsy patients and comparison to 151 previously reported necropsy patients.* Am Heart J 1982, 104: 115-25.

74. Recchia, D., Sharkey, A.M., Bosner, M.S., Kouchoukos, N.T., Nickline, S.A. *Sensitive detection of abnormal aortic architecture in Marfan syndrome with high-frequency ultrasonic tissue characterization.* Circulation 1995, 91: 1036-43.

75. Thiene, G., Basso, C., Danieli, G.A., Rampazzo, A., Corrado, D., Nava, A. *Arrhythmogenic right ventricular cardiomyopathy: A still under-recognized clinical entity.* Trends Cardiovasc Med 1997, 7: 84-90.

76. Legislation of October 26, 1971. *Tutela sanitaria delle attività sportive (medical protection of athletic activities).* Gazzetta Ufficiale, December 23, 1971: 8162-4.

77. Decree of the Italian Ministry of Health, February 18, 1982. *Norme per la tutela sanitaria dell'attività sportiva agonistica (rules concerning the medical protection of athletic activity).* Gazzetta Ufficiale, March 5, 1982: 1715-9.

78. Maron, B.J., Thompson, P.D., Puffer, J.C., et al. *Cardiovascular preparticipation screening of competitive athletes. A statement for health professionals from the sudden death committee (clinical cardiology) and congenital cardiac defects committee (cardiovascular disease in the young), American Heart Association.* Circulation 1996, 94: 850-6.

79. Maron, B.J., Mitchell, J.H. *26th Bethesda Conference: Recommendations for detecting eligibility for competition in athletes with cardiovascular abnormalities.* J Am Coll Cardiol 1994, 24: 845-99.

CHAPTER 6

MARKERS AND TRIGGERS OF SUDDEN DEATH IN ATHLETES

M.T. Subirana[1], R. Elosua[2], X. Viñolas[1], P. Ferrés[1], T. Bayés-Genís[1],
J. Guindo[1], T. Martínez-Rubio[1] and A. Bayés de Luna[1]
[1]Department of Cardiology and Cardiac Surgery, Hospital de la Santa
Creu i Sant Pau, Barcelona and [2]Lipids and Cardiovascular
Epidemiology Unit, Institut Municipal d'Investigació Mèdica, Barcelona.

The markers and triggers of sudden death in the general population have been well studied (1-3). In principle, they are related to the presence of a vulnerable myocardium in which some triggers or modulators may induce sudden death, generally through ventricular fibrillation (VF) (Fig. 1). Ventricular fibrillation may be triggered by a single event, as happens with a sustained ventricular tachycardia during a waterfall (Fig. 2) or by a more complex cascade of events (Fig. 3). Sometimes the final step is a bradyarrhythmia. This is relatively frequent in patients with advanced congestive heart failure (4) but is rare in the ambulatory sudden death of patients with different types of heart disease (5) and in the acute phase of myocardial infarction (6) (Fig. 4).

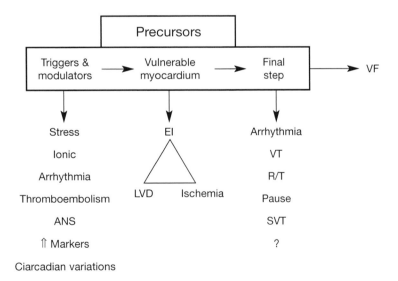

Figure 1. Precursors of sudden death due to ventricular fibrillation. These included triggers and modulators, markers of vulnerable myocardium and the final arrhythmia. VF: ventricular fibrillation; VT: ventricular tachycardia; EI: electrical instability; LVD: left ventricular dysfunction; SVT: sustained ventricular tachycardia; ANS: autonomous nervous system.

A. Bayés de Luna et al. (eds.), Arrhythmias and Sudden Death in Athletes, 71–88.

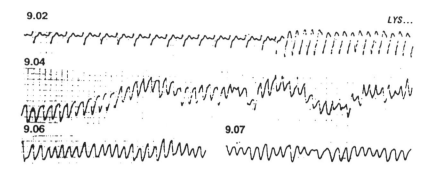

Figure 2. Ventricular fibrillation triggered by a sustained ventricular tachycardia.

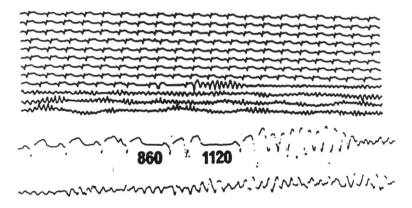

Figure 3. Cascade of events (premature atrial complex, pause, normal beat, premature ventricular complex (PVC), longer pause, normal beat, R/T PVC) that finally ends in a ventricular fibrillation.

Sudden death is very rare in athletes. Its incidence ranges between 0.75 and 0.13 per 100,000 in young male and female athletes and is 6 per 100,000 in middle-aged men per year (7, 8). Most of these catastrophic events are related to a cardiovascular abnormality (9). The need for cardiovascular preparticipation screening in athletes to prevent sudden death has been defined and established (10). Evidently, if good periodic screening before competitive sports had been performed, some of these deaths might have been avoided due to the detection of abnormalities. Competitive sport, therefore, would have not been recommended. How to perform the screening and its different steps are discussed in chapter 7.

In this chapter we will review and comment on the most important markers and triggers of sudden death in athletes who, in general, do not present previous evident heart disease.

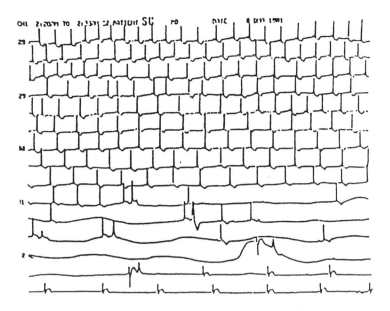

Figure 4. Progressive bradyarrhythmia as the final step before sudden death in a patient with acute myocardial infarction and electromechanical dissociation.

Markers of Sudden Death in Athletes

In principle, sudden death does not appear in the absence of a vulnerable myocardium. This means that in the majority of cases of sudden death (>90%) we may find, after careful screening, some evidence of heart disease. Nevertheless, using current diagnostic procedures, we are unable to find any evidence in a few cases (11). However, very probably the abnormality exists in the form of a localized left ventricular hypertrophy, subtle abnormalities of repolarization, an imbalance of the autonomic nervous system (ANS), undetected previous myocarditis or ultrasilent myocardial ischemia.

The most frequent triggers of sudden death and markers of vulnerable myocardium, usually silent, in athletes at risk of sudden death are shown in Table 1. We will comment on the most important characteristics of all of them.

MARKERS OF PATHOLOGICAL LEFT VENTRICULAR HYPERTROPHY: ATHLETE'S HEART *VERSUS* HYPERTROPHIC CARDIOMYOPATHY

Left ventricular hypertrophy (LVH) is, in some circumstances, a useful physiological adaptive mechanism although in others it represents an evident pathological process. The most characteristic type of pathological LVH is found in patients with hypertrophic cardiomyopathy (HCM). In HCM, and probably related to a specific type of left ventricular disarray, the incidence of ventricular arrhythmias and sudden death is high (12). The differential diagnosis between physiological and pathological hypertrophy in athletes is very important (13) and every effort to try to clarify this problem should be welcomed.

Table 1. Triggers of sudden death and markers of vulnerable myocardium in athletes at risk of sudden death.

Triggers	Markers of VM	Final event
1. Physical and /or psychological stress 2. Appearance of a paroxysmal arrhythmia 3. Brusque ANS imbalance 4. Crisis of ischemia	1. LVH: HCM 2. IHD 3. Electrical instability 4. Presence of other heart disease 5. Genetic markers 6. Idiopathic arrhythmia substrate: SVT/VF.	Usually due to VF and during exercise

ANS: autonomous nervous system; VM: vulnerable myocardium; LVH: left ventricular hypertrophy; HCM: hypertrophic cardiomyopathy; IHD: ischemic heart disease; SVT: sustained ventricular tachycardia; VF: ventricular fibrillation.

It is necessary to establish the criteria that allow us to differentiate between physiological LVH and HCM. Some parameters, according to Maron *et al.* (13), that may be useful in establishing the differential diagnosis and in decreasing the gray area between both processes are presented in Figure 5. Briefly, HCM would be supported by the following data: i) the presence of an unusual pattern of left ventricular hypertrophy on echocardiography; ii) an end diastolic left ventricular diameter <45 mm; iii) left atrial enlargement; iv) bizarre electrocardiographic patterns; v) abnormal left ventricular filling pattern; vi) female gender; vii) lack of decrease in left ventricular thickness with deconditioning and viii) family history of HCM.

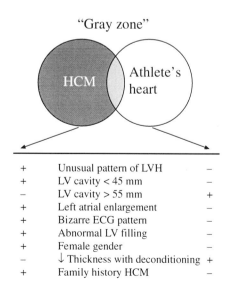

Figure 5. Criteria used to distinguish hypertrophic cardiomyopathy (HCM) from athlete's heart when the left ventricular (LV) wall thickness is within the gray zone of overlap, consistent with both diagnoses. Adapted from reference 13.

In some cases it is still very difficult to differentiate between these two types of LVH, in spite of all these parameters. In our opinion, there are different new possibilities that could help us to make a differential diagnosis and consequently would allow us to reduce the gray area.

For a better study of LVH characteristics, we have to consider that cardiac muscle is much more than myocyte mass and, as a consequence, we have to study not only myocytes but also the other cardiac mass components: interstitium, microvasculature and autonomic innervation (14) (Fig. 6). We will comment on our noninvasive approach to studying these different components (Table 2). We are not considering invasive techniques (electrophysiology, biopsy, hemodynamic studies, etc.) or some noninvasive techniques that are not usually available, such as positron emission tomography.

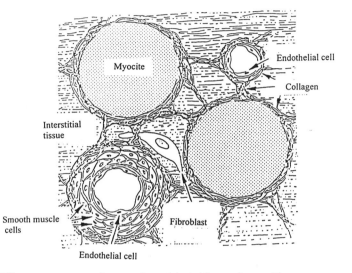

Figure 6. Different components of myocardium. Adapted from reference 14.

Table 2. Noninvasive approach to study the different components of ventricular mass.

Components of ventricular mass	Noninvasive methods to study each component
Myocyte mass and integrity	Echocardiography
	Magnetic resonance image
	Antimyosin uptake
	Genetic
Ventricular function	Echocardiography
	Nuclear medicine
Interstitial fibrosis	Ultrasonic myocardial reflection
	Serum concentration of procollagen
	Late potentials
Microcirculation	Exercise testing
	Nuclear medicine
Impairment of autonomous nervous system	Repolarization study (QT dispersion, QT dynamic behavior, T-wave alternans, ...)
	Heart rate variability
	Nuclear techniques (MIBG)

Myocyte Mass: Anatomic, Ultrastructural and Functional Aspects
Echocardiography is considered the gold standard for the study of ventricular mass and size. According to Pelliccia *et al.* (15), the upper physiological limit of left ventricular thickness is 12.9 mm. Thus, the detection of a left ventricular wall thickness of or greater than 13 mm, except perhaps in rowers, canoeists and possibly cyclists, should be considered abnormal.

Magnetic resonance imaging (MRI), however, allows all segments of the left ventricle to be studied in greater detail. We studied 30 patients with HCM and found that with echocardiography we could assess only 67% of all left ventricular segments, while with MRI we were able to assess 97% of them (16). Furthermore, with echocardiography we were able to assess all left ventricular segments in only 27% of patients with HCM whereas with MRI we could assess all left ventricular segments in 77% of the patients (16). In Figure 7 we present a case that may be used as an example of this. Thus, it is clear that MRI may increase the potential to detect left ventricular hypertrophy, especially localized forms, and thus may play a role in the diagnosis of this pathology.

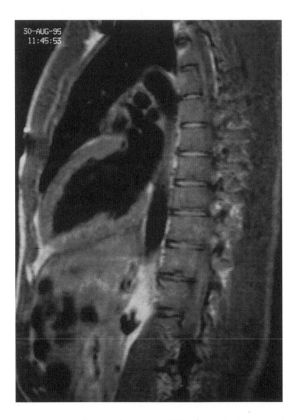

Figure 7. A cardiac magnetic resonance image of an athlete (23 years old) with a positive exercise test but with normal coronary arteries, showing a localized left ventricular hypertrophy in the basal segment of the septum.

To study myocyte integrity it may be useful to determine antimyosin antibody uptake. Monoclonal 111 Indium-labeled antimyosin antibodies are fixed by myocardial cells when the membrane ruptures. This technique is very sensitive but has low specificity in evaluating myocardial damage and has been used to study myocarditis, dilated cardiomyopathy, myocardial infarction and heart transplant rejection (17-20). There is also evidence of a high prevalence of positive Indium-labeled antimyosin uptake after radiofrequency ablation (21). We studied antimyosin antibody uptake in a group of athletes with a wall thickness greater than 11 mm and in a group of patients with HCM and a wall thickness greater than 13 mm (22). Sixty-four percent of athletes presented a positive antimyosin uptake, with a mean heart-to-lung ratio of 1.59 (normal <1.56). On the other hand, all the patients with HCM presented positive antimyosin uptake with a heart-to-lung ratio mean value of 1.77 (22) (Fig. 8). Most of the athletes with positive antimyosin uptake performed well. As the real importance and meaning of this finding is at the moment unclear, we do not consider that such athletes should stop practicing sport. It is clear however, that it is advisable to follow-up their medical history carefully.

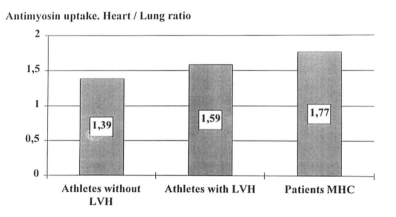

Figure 8. Mean antimyosin uptake in athletes without left ventricular hypertrophy, in athletes with left ventricular hypertrophy (LVH) and in patients with hypertrophic cardiomyopathy (HCM).

Regarding ventricular function, systolic and diastolic function may be studied. It is interesting to consider the behavior of systolic function during exercise. There is some evidence that the basal ejection fraction of top ranking athletes is not higher than that found in sedentary people (23, 24) and what is more striking is that in some cases the ejection fraction does not increase during exercise (25). Some explanations exist for this phenomenon but none of them give provides a clear answer to this, in principle, strange behavior.

Concerning diastolic function, there is evidence that interstitial fibrosis is responsible for its impairment. This has been proved in hemodynamic studies (26) and may clearly be shown by endomyocardial biopsy. There are, however, other noninvasive ways to study it (see below).

Interstitium

Ultrasonic myocardial reflectivity is a relatively new echocardiographic technique that allows us to obtain an index of the collagen content in patients with LVH (27). It has been demonstrated that athletes with the same degree of LVH as patients with HCM present a normal reflectivity, whereas patients with HCM present a higher reflectivity that expresses an increased myocardium collagen content (Fig. 9) (28). Thus, this technique may help us to differentiate athletes with physiological LVH from patients with HCM, both of whom present a similar degree of left ventricular wall thickness.

The presence of fibrosis may also be suspected if we demonstrate an increase of serum concentration of procollagen III amino-terminal peptide and procollagen I carboxy-terminal peptide, which are markers of collagen III synthesis. Diez *et al.* (29) have demonstrated that in patients with LVH due to systemic hypertension, and without any evidence

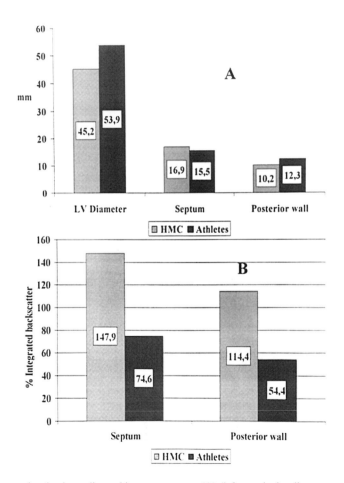

Figure 9. Conventional echocardiographic measurements (A) (left ventricular diameter and wall thickness) and the quantitative ultrasound data (B) (% integrated backscatter) of myocardial structures in a group of patients with hypertrophic cardiomyopathy and a group of athletes with similar values of wall thickness.

of other systemic disease which could be related to interstitial fibrosis, the serum concentration of these collagen peptides is very high and decreases after treatment with drugs that reduce fibrosis, such as angiotensin-converting enzyme inhibitors (Fig. 10). The same authors have also demonstrated a relationship between the number and characteristics of premature ventricular complex according to Lown's classification and the serum concentration of procollagen type I (Table 3). Furthermore, these authors (30) have observed that there is a clear relationship between the degree of interstitial fibrosis found in the heart muscle of spontaneously hypertensive rats and the level of serum concentration in procollagen. Although it is speculative to consider that these measurements may be useful in separating physiological from pathological hypertrophy, this is another way to try to solve this problem.

Theoretically, the positivity of late potentials may also be related to interstitial fibrosis (31). We know, at least, that positive late potentials are more prevalent in patients with

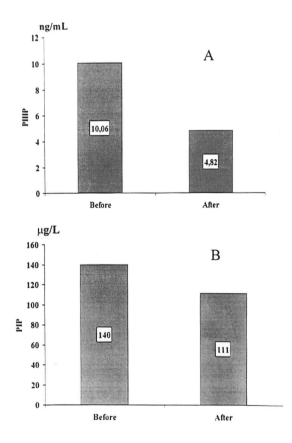

Figure 10. Serum concentration of procollagen type III amino terminal peptide (PIIIP) (A) and of procollagen type I carboxy terminal peptide (PIP) (B) in essential hypertensive patients before and after treatment with lisinopril. Adapted from reference 29.

HCM than in athletes with LVH. Furthermore, athletes with LVH and late potentials frequently present inducibility of nonsustained ventricular tachycardia in electrophysiologic studies (32).

Table 3. Serum concentrations (mean ± standard error) of procollagen type III amino terminal peptide (PIIIP) and procollagen type I carboxy terminal peptide (PIP) in hypertensive patients according to Lown-Wolf's classification of ventricular arrhythmias. Adapted from (29).

Lown grade	0	1	2	3
Number of patients	12	25	9	4
PIIIP (ng/ml)	9.95 ± 0.83	10.63 ± 0.68	9.86 ± 0.99	9.59 ± 2.54
PIP (µg/l)	121 ± 7	130 ± 7	144 ± 10	179 ± 25

Microcirculation

There are different ways of explaining alterations in the microcirculation of patients with LVH (33). Iriarte *et al.* (34) found that angina in patients with systemic hypertension and left ventricular hypertrophy is frequently associated with microvascular disease. They have also shown that after enalapril treatment, angina frequently disappears and scintigraphy also normalizes as a consequence of improvement in microcirculation, probably related to hypertrophy decrease. There is some evidence that exhaustive training may also induce a ventricular mass/capillary network imbalance that may be responsible for microvascular ischemia.

Nevertheless, the role of alterations in microcirculation and arrhythmia has not been well defined.

Autonomous Nervous System

Impairment of the ANS may be studied in different ways, which may help, at least theoretically, to differentiate between physiological and pathological hypertrophy. In surface ECG the study of QT dispersion may provide some information to stratify risk in athletes with ventricular arrhythmia (32).

Nevertheless, it is with Holter technology that we are able to further determine ANS impairment, especially with the study of heart rate variability (35, 36) and QT dynamics (37-40). The results of these studies with linear standard techniques (time and frequency domain) in different subsets of patients are well known. Furthermore, different nonlinear techniques that include 3D Poincare plots and entropy have recently been described (41, 42). Nevertheless, its usefulness in differentiating physiological from pathological LVH needs to be validated.

Another technique for studying ANS is the uptake of MIBG (I 123 meta-iodobenzylguanidine) an analog of guanidine by the sympathetic nerves in the same way as noradrenaline (43, 44). Lack of uniformity in the uptake of MIBG identifies regional defects in cardiac sympathetic innervation. This has been demonstrated in patients who have had a myocardial infarction (45) and in those with malignant ventricular arrhythmia (46). We wonder whether this technique could be used to study ANS imbalance but again, its value in differentiating physiological from pathological LVH remains to be proved.

MARKERS OF ISCHEMIA

Ischemic heart disease (IHD) is the most frequent cause of sudden death in athletes older than 35 years and is the second cause of sudden death in athletes younger than 35 (9). Thus, the presence of repolarization abnormalities in surface ECG, exercise ECG or precordial pain gives rise to a possible diagnosis of IHD. In these cases other complementary tests, including coronariography, are mandatory in order to confirm the diagnosis if necessary.

The use of an exercise test as a screening technique in athletes older than 35 years is under discussion. The current guidelines do not recommend the exercise test in asymptomatic athletes (10). The prevalence of a positive exercise test in competitive athletes is low and even its positivity is usually not related to any evidence of coronary atherosclerosis.

We have demonstrated that athletes with very abnormal repolarization in surface electrocardiogram (ECG) and without any evidence of HCM from echocardiography do not present abnormalities suggestive of ischemia by isotopic studies (47).

A new noninvasive technique that may be useful in the diagnosis of IHD is ultrafast scanner tomography (48). If this test is negative, which means absent or low calcium deposits in the coronary arteries, the possibility of coronary stenosis is very low.

In athletes with symptoms suggestive of angina, it is also important to determine the presence of coronary risk factors, especially dyslipemia, smoking and hypertension.

Another possible explanation for the presence in athletes of ischemia and malignant arrhythmia unrelated to atherosclerosis is the evidence of a milking (49) or a cardiac vasospasm (50). Furthermore, alterations of microcirculation may also be involved (see above).

MARKERS OF ELECTRICAL INSTABILITY

In chapter 7 the most important arrhythmias and their relevance to sports performance are described. We will discuss some noninvasive markers of electrical instability in athletes and focus on the role of surface ECG to detect this potential instability.

Wolf-Parkinson-White syndrome can be diagnosed. Different invasive and noninvasive risk markers in this syndrome have been described (51, 52). Surface ECG usually detects preexcitation but sometimes this is intermittent or even completely canceled. In all athletes with palpitations it is compulsory to try to identify the arrhythmia responsible with electrophysiologic study if necessary and, if the anatomical substrate of arrhythmia is identified, radiofrequency ablation is recommended.

Several risk markers in long QT syndrome have also been identified (53, 54). Recently, Brugada *et al.* (55) have described the morphology of right bundle-branch block and precordial injury pattern in V1 through V3 as an arrhythmogenic marker that identifies patients at high risk of ventricular fibrillation or sudden death. The same observation has been documented in another study (56).

Surface ECG can be also useful in suspecting arrhythmogenic right ventricle dysplasia. This cardiomyopathy has been considered as a disease associated with young patients who die suddenly (57, 58). The diagnosis of right ventricular dysplasia is based on echocardiography, although an abnormal ECG may be useful in suggesting the diagnosis (59, 60).

In the surface ECG it is also possible to measure QT dispersion, which is a marker of electrical instability (61) and has been used to stratify risk in different substrates of patients.

There are, as has already been mentioned, many other electrocardiological techniques (Holter technology, T-wave alternans techniques, signal averaged electrocardiography (62), etc.) that may be used to detect electrical instability and to study abnormalities of the ANS. These may help to stratify risk in different substrates of patients. The value of these techniques as a marker of electrical instability in athletes needs to be clarified.

PRESENCE OF OTHER HEART DISEASES
Although the majority of deaths in competitive athletes occur in the presence of HCM, IHD or electrical instability, on some occasions they may occur in the presence of other heart diseases that have not been diagnosed in the previous screening: mild dilated cardiomyopathy, arrhythmogenic right ventricular dysplasia, congenital abnormalities and mitral valve prolapse, among others.

GENETIC MARKERS
Several mutations in different genes have been shown to cause certain diseases: hypertrophic cardiomyopathy (63), long QT syndrome (64) and arrhythmogenic right ventricular cardiomyopathy (65). These mutations are still a research procedure and they are not routinely used in clinical cardiology; however, some of these mutations have been associated with prognosis, especially in the case of hypertrophic cardiomyopathy (66). Mutations in genes coding for the β-myosin heavy chain (β-MyHC), cardiac troponin T (cTnT), cardiac troponin I, α-tropomyosin, myosin binding protein C (MyBP-C) and myosin light chains 1 and 2 have been identified as being responsible for different types of hypertrophic cardiomyopathy. In the β-MyHC protein gene, the Gly256Glu, Val-606Met and Leu908Val mutations are associated with a benign prognosis, whereas Arg403Gln, Arg719Trp and Arg543Cys mutations are associated with a high incidence of sudden death. Mutations in the cTnT protein gene are associated with mild hypertrophy but also with a high incidence of sudden death. Mutations in MyBP-C are associated with mild hypertrophy and a benign prognosis.

Nevertheless, there are other factors besides genetics (environmental factors and their interaction with genetics) that modulate phenotypic expression and prognosis of hypertrophic cardiomyopathy.

IDIOPATHIC VENTRICULAR FIBRILLATION
Even with the recent descriptions of new diseases (Brugada syndrome, etc.) in some sudden deaths among athletes no abnormal structural or functional heart disease can be found with currently available techniques. We therefore classify these deaths as idiopathic (or primary) ventricular fibrillation when all possible causes (see above) have been ruled out. The data regarding the follow-up in this very infrequent situation are collected in the unexplained cardiac arrest registry of Europe (11). At the moment we know that a new episode of ventricular fibrillation occurs in at least 40% of the patients, even if symptom-free periods of months or years are observed. No antiarrhythmic drug seems to

effectively prevent a new episode of ventricular fibrillation and the implantation of an automatic defibrillator, plus cessation of sports activity is recommended. A close follow-up is needed in order to rule out the development of an organic heart disease (especially right ventricular dysplasia or masked Brugada syndrome) in the future. Genetic data are not currently available but in future could perhaps help us to understand the underlying mechanism of this mysterious disease.

Triggers of Sudden Death

There is evidence that some triggers may precipitate malignant arrhythmia that leads to ventricular fibrillation and sudden death. In athletes this syndrome usually presents itself during exercise although exceptionally it may appear during rest. What the final triggers are remains uncertain but there is some evidence to suggest possible causes, which we discuss below.

PHYSICAL AND MENTAL STRESS

Some observations suggest the importance of physical or mental stress in triggering sudden death (67). The frequencies of onset of sudden death, as well as myocardial infarction, show a marked circadian rhythm with a marked morning increase. Transient myocardial ischemia shows a similar morning increase. Ruptured atherosclerotic plaque lies at the base of coronary thrombosis and mental or physical stress can cause a plaque rupture. Some physiologic processes leading to plaque rupture (hypercoagulability, vasoconstriction) are accentuated in the morning.

In 1993 Mitlleman *et al.* and Willich *et al.* (68, 69) reported that exercise could be considered a trigger of myocardial infarction. The risk of presenting a myocardial infarction is increased during exercise and one hour after. One important consideration is that habitual vigorous exercise is associated with an overall decreased risk of myocardial infarction (Fig. 12). The same conclusion was observed by Siscovick *et al.* (70) who concluded that the risk of primary cardiac arrest is transiently increased during vigorous exercise, mainly in sedentary people (Fig. 11).

Exercise may also be a trigger of sudden death in patients with long QT syndrome and in some sympathetic-related malignant ventricular arrhythmias.

The cellular mechanism involved in the relation between exercise and sudden death may be also explained by ionic disturbances. During exercise K^+ is released from contracting skeletal muscle, which results in an exercise-induced hyperkalemia that is mainly dependent on exercise intensity and the physical fitness of the individual. During the recovery period, a rapid decrease in plasma $[K^+]$ is observed. These rapid increases and decreases in plasma $[K^+]$ related to exercise onset and cessation have been implicated in altered myocardial function and sudden death (71).

DRUGS

Before carrying out any medical investigation to diagnose an arrhythmogenic substrate, a careful clinical history must be obtained. At this point, it is very important to record the

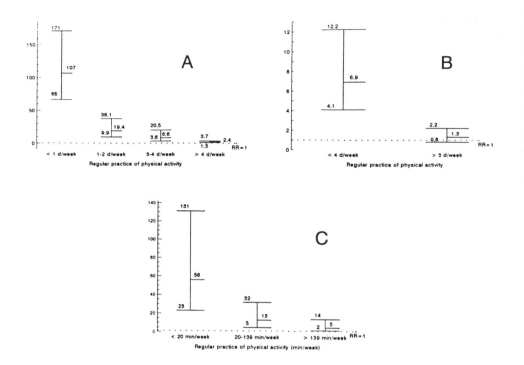

Figure 11. Relative risk of acute myocardial infarction (A and B) or sudden death (C) during heavy physical activity practice (intensity > 6 METs) in different groups according to regular practice of physical activity. Adapted from references 67-69.

use and abuse of drugs. Some common drugs can trigger a malignant ventricular arrhythmia: quinidine, phenothiazines, erythromycin and other macrolides, as well as antihistaminic drugs (72, 73).

The link between alcohol and sudden death has not been conclusively demonstrated although some studies have reported that lethal ventricular arrhythmias may precede alcoholic cardiomyopathy (74). On the other hand, cocaine is a drug with adverse cardiovascular effects, which are dependent on the dose, rate of administration and duration of use. Cocaine is a powerful sympathomimetic drug that lowers the threshold for coronary vasoconstriction, myocardial ischemia and infarction; moreover, cocaine causes autonomic disturbances and alters catecholamine homeostasis (75).

SUPRAVENTRICULAR ARRHYTHMIA
In patients with Wolf-Parkinson-White syndrome, the rare cases of ventricular fibrillation are usually triggered by a rapid atrial fibrillation, sometimes produced by exercise.

BRUSQUE AUTONOMIC NERVOUS SYSTEM IMBALANCE
Although there is no evidence in athletes, a sudden excess of heart rate variability and QT length may be present before malignant ventricular arrhythmias.

CRISIS OF ISCHEMIA
Crisis of ischemia are not frequent in athletes. Nevertheless, even in the absence of atherosclerotic heart disease, the presence of coronary artery spasms or myocardial bridges may be related to a crisis of sudden ischemia that may be potentially dangerous.

COMMOTIO CORDIS
Sudden death may occur during the practice of sport after a blunt blow to the chest, in spite of a normal heart. The impact does not need to be very strong and in Maron *et al.*'s report (76) on 25 children and young adults (age: 3 to 19 years) who collapsed after an unexpected blow to the chest, 28% were wearing some type of precordial protection. Link *et al.* (77) have demonstrated that the cause of sudden death was a ventricular fibrillation induced by the abrupt precordial blow, being delivered in the vulnerable phase of ventricular excitability.

Final Event

Sudden death in athletes is very rare and consequently it is very difficult to determine the final event before death in this population. In some subsets of patients this has been demonstrated more easily because there is more evidence of sudden death while wearing a Holter device. In acute myocardial infarction the most frequent final event is primary ventricular tachycardia. In patients with advanced heart disease it is ventricular tachycardia leading to ventricular fibrillation. However, in patients with advanced heart failure the most frequent final event is severe bradyarrhythmia.

In the case of sudden death in athletes, the evidence is much scarcer but there are some data that support the idea that the final event is ventricular fibrillation sometimes preceded by ventricular tachycardia. This is probably what happens most frequently in patients with HCM. However in patients with Wolf-Parkinson-White syndrome or in athletes without evidence of any heart disease, there is evidence that primary ventricular fibrillation is the cause of sudden death.

References

1. Myerburg, R.J., Castellanos, A. *Cardiac arrest and sudden cardiac death*. In: Heart Disease. E. Braunwald (Ed.). WB Saunders Company: Philadelphia 1997, 742-79.
2. Bayés-Genís, A., Viñolas, X., Guindo, J., Fiol, M., Bayés de Luna, A. *Electrocardiographic and clinical precursors of ventricular fibrillation: Chain of events*. J Cardiovasc Electrophysiol 1995, 6: 410-7.
3. Goldstein, S., Bayés de Luna, A., Guindo Soldevila, J. Sudden Cardiac Death. Futura Publishing Company, Inc.: Armonk, New York 1994.
4. Luu, M., Stevenson, W.G., Stevenson, L.W., Baron, K., Walden, J. *Diverse mechanism of unexpected cardiac arrest in advanced heart failures*. Circulation 1988, 80: 1675-80.
5. Bayés de Luna, A., Coumel, P., Leclercq, J.F. *Ambulatory sudden death: Mechanism of production of fatal arrhythmia syndromes on the bases of data from 157 cases*. Am Heart J 1989, 117: 151-9.
6. Adgey, A.A., Devlin, J.E., Webb, S.W., Mulholland, H.C. *Initiation of ventricular fibrillation outside hospital in patients with acute ischemic heart disease*. Br Heart J 1982, 47: 55-6.

7.   Thompson, P.D. *The cardiovascular complications of vigorous physical activity.* Arch Intern Med 1996, 156: 2297-302.
8.   Kohl, H.W. III, Powell, K.E., Gordon, N.F., Blair, S.N., Paffenbarger, R.S. *Physical activity, physical fitness and sudden cardiac death.* Epidemiol Rev 1992, 14: 37-58.
9.   Maron, B.J., Shirani, J., Poliac, L.C., Mathenge, R., Roberts, W.C., Mueeler, F.O. *Sudden death in young competitive athletes. Clinical, demographic, and pathological profiles.* JAMA 1996, 276(3): 199-204.
10. Maron, B.J., Thompson, P.D., Puffer, J.C., et al. *Cardiovascular preparticipation screening of competitive athletes. A statement for health professionals from the Sudden Death Committee (clinical cardiology) and Congenital Cardiac Defects Committee (cardiovascular disease in the young). American Heart Association.* Circulation 1996, 94(4): 850-6.
11. Consensus Statement of the Joint Steering Committees of the Unexplained Cardiac Arrest Registry of Europe and of the Idiopathic Ventricular Fibrillation Registry of the United States. *Survivors of out-of-hospital cardiac arrest with apparently normal heart.* Circulation 1997, 95: 265-72.
12. McKenna, W., Deanfield, J., Faruqui, A., England, D., Oakley, C.M., Goodwin, J.F. *Prognosis in hypertrophic cardiomyopathy: Role of age and clinical and hemodynamic features.* Am J Cardiol 1981, 47:532-8.
13. Maron, B.J., Pelliccia, A., Spirito, P. *Cardiac disease in young trained athletes. Insights into methods for distinguishing athlete's heart from structural heart disease, with particular emphasis on hypertrophic cardiomyopathy.* Circulation 1995, 91: 1596-601.
14. Weber, K.T., Brilla, C.G. *Pathological hypertrophy and cardiac interstitium. Fibrosis and renin-angiotensin-aldosterone system.* Circulation 1991, 83: 1849-65.
15. Pelliccia, A., Maron, B.J., Spataro, A., Proschan, M.A., Spirito, P. *The upper limit of physiologic cardiac hypertrophy in highly trained elite athletes.* New Engl J Med 1991, 324: 295-301.
16. Pons-Lladó, G., Carreras, F., Borrás, X., Palmer, J., Llauger, J., Bayés de Luna, A. *Comparison of morphological assessment of hypertrophic cardiomyopathy by magnetic resonance versus echocardiographic imaging.* Am J Cardiol 1997, 79: 1651-6.
17. Yasuda, T., Palacios, I.F., Dec, G.W., et al. *Indium 111-monoclonal antimyosin antibody imaging in the diagnosis of acute myocarditis.* Circulation 1987, 76: 306-11.
18. Obrador, D., Ballester, M., Carió, I., Bernà, L., Pons-Lladó, G. *High prevalence of myocardial monoclonal antimyosin antibody uptake in patients with chronic dilated cardiomyopathy.* J Am Coll Cadiol 1989, 13: 1289-93.
19. Khaw, B.A., Gold, H.K., Yasuda, T. *Scintigraphic quantification of myocardial necrosis in patients after intravenous injection of myosin-specific antibody.* Circulation 1986, 74: 501-8.
21. Ballester, M., Obrador, D., Carrió, I., et al. *Early postoperative reduction of monoclonal antimyosin antibody uptake is associated with absent rejection-related complications after heart transplantation.* Circulation 1992, 85: 61-8.
21. Viñolas, X., Carrió, I., Oter, R., et al. *Evaluation of myocardial lesion after radiofrequency catheter ablation using In-111-antimyosin antibody prospective study.* New Trends Arrhythmias 1995, 9: 745.
22. Subirana, M.T., Ferrés, P., Elosua, R., et al. *111-In-antimyosin antibody uptake in athletes with left ventricular hypertrophy.* Eur Heart J 1997, 18: 252 (Abstract).
23. Rerych, S.K., Scholz, P.M., Sabiston, D.C., Jones, R.H. *Effects of exercise training on left ventricular function in normal subjects: A longitudinal study by radionuclide angiography.* Am J Cardiol 1980, 45: 244-52.
24. Fagard, R., Aubert, A., Lysens, R., Staessens, S., Vanhees, L., Amery, A. *Non-invasive assessment of seasonal variations in cardiac structure and function in cyclists.* Circulation 1983, 67: 896-901.
25. Fisman, E.Z., Frank, A.G., Ben-Ari, E., et al. *Altered left volume and ejection fraction responses to supine dynamic exercise in athletes.* J Am Coll Cardiol 1990, 15: 582-8.
26. Hess, O.M., Schneider, J., Koch, R., Bamert, C., Grimm, J., Krayenbuehl, H.P. *Diastolic function and myocardial structure in patients with myocardial hypertrophy. Special reference to normalized viscoelastic data.* Circulation 1981, 63: 360-71.
27. Skorton, D.J. *Noninvasive assessment of myocardial composition and function in the hypertrophied heart.* Circulation 1989, 80: 1095-7.
28. Lattanzi, F., Di Bello, V., Picano, E., et al. *Normal ultrasonic myocardial reflectivity in athletes with increased left ventricular mass. A tissue characterization study.* Circulation 1992, 85: 1828-34.
29. Diez, J., Laviades, C., Mayor, G., Gil, M.J., Monreal, I. *Increased serum concentrations of procollagen peptides in essential hypertension. Relation to cardiac alterations.* Circulation 1995, 91: 1450-6.

30. Díez, J., Panizo, A., Gil, M.J., Monreal, I., Hernández, M., Pardo-Mindán, J. *Serum markers of collagen type I metabolism in spontaneuously hypertensive rats. Relation to myocardial fibrosis.* Circulation 1996, 93: 1026-32.
31. Mehta, D., McKenna, W., Ward, D.E., Davies, M.J., Camm, A.J. *Significance of signal-averaged electrocardiography in relation to endomyocardial biopsy and ventricular stimulation studies in patients with ventricular tachycardia without clinically apparent heart disease.* J Am Coll Cardiol 1989, 14: 372-9.
32. Jordaens, L., Missault, L., Pelleman, G., Duprez, D., Backer, G.D., Clement, D.L. *Comparison of athletes with life-threateing ventricular arrhythmias with two groups of healthy athletes and a group of normal control subjects.* Am J Cardiol 1994, 74: 1124-8.
33. Kaski, J.C. Angina Pectoris with Normal Coronary Arteries. Sindrome X. Kluwer Academic Publishers: Boston 1995.
34. Iriate, M.M., Caso, R., Murga, N., López de Argumedo, M., Sagastagoitia, D. *Microvascular angina in systemic hypertension: Diagnosis and treatment with enalapril.* Am J Cardiol 1995, 76: 31-4.
35. Kleiger, R.E., Miller, J.P., Bigger, J.T., et al. *Decreased heart rate variability and its association with increased mortality after acute myocardial infarction.* Am J Cardiol 1987, 59: 256-62.
36. Camm, J., Fei, L. *Clinical significance of heart rate variability.* In: Noninvasive Electrocardiology. Clinical Aspects of Holter monitoring. A.J. Moss, S. Stern (Eds.). W.B. Saunders Company Ltd.: London 1996, 225-48.
37. Marti, V., Guindo, J., Homs, E., Viñolas, X., Bayés de Luna, A. *Peaks of QTc lengthening in Holter recording as a marker of life-threatening arrhythmias in postmyocardial infarction patients.* Am Heart J 1992, 124: 234-5.
38. Homs, E., Martí, V., Guindo, J., et al. *Automatic measurement of corrected QT interval in Holter recordings: Comparison of its dynamic behavior in postmyocardial infarction patients with and without life threatening arrhythmias.* Am Heart J 1997, 134 (Suppl. 2 Pt.1): 181-7.
39. Laguna, P., Thakor, N.V., Caminal, P., et al. *New algorithm for QT interval analysis in 24-hour Holter ECG: Performance and applications.* Med Biol Eng Comput 1990, 28: 67-73.
40. Viñolas, X., Bayés-Genis, A., Guindo, J., et al. *Circadian repolarization patterns and ventricular arrhythmias.* In: Noninvasive Electrocardiology. Clinical Aspects of Holter Monitoring. A.J. Moss, S. Stern (Eds.). W.B. Saunders Company Ltd.: London 1996, 479-91.
41. Zebrowski, J.J., Poplawska, W., Baranowski, R., Buchner, T. *Local time properties of 24-hour holter recordings RR intervals: A nonlinear quantitative method through patterns entropy of 3-D return maps.* Computers in Cardiology 1995, 377-80.
42. Baranowski, R., Zebrowski, J.J., Poplawska, W., et al. *3-Dimensional poincare plots of the QT intervals –an approach to nonlinear QT analysis.* Computers in Cardiology 1995, 789-92.
43. Wieland, D.W., Brown, L.E., Rogers, W.L., et al. *Myocardial imaging with a radioiodinated norepinephrine storage analog.* J Nucl Med 1981, 22: 22-31.
44. Kline, R.C., Swanson, D.P., Wieland, D.M., et al. *Myocardial imaging in man with I-123 metaiodobenzylguanidine.* J Nucl Med 1981, 22: 129-32.
45. Stanton, M.S., Tuli, M.M., Radtke, N.L., et al. *Regional sympathetic denervation after myocardial infarction in humans detected noninvasively using I-123-metaiodobenzylguanidine.* J Am Coll Cardiol 1989, 14: 1519-26.
46. Casses-Senon, D., Philippe, L., Cosnay, P., et al. *Etude isotopique de la perfusion et de l'innervation myocardique chez 28 patients atteints de cardiomyopathie hypertrophique primitive: Relation avec les troubles du rythme ventriculaire.* Arch Mal Coeur 1994, 87: 475-83.
47. Serra-Grima, J.S., Carrió, I., Estorch, M., et al. *ECG alterations in the athlete type "pseudoischemia".* J Sports Card 1986, 3: 9-16.
48. Budoff, M.J., Georgiou, D., Brody, A., et al. *Ultrafast computer tomography as a diagnostic modality in the detection of coronary artery disease: A multicenter study.* Circulation 1996, 93(5): 898-904.
49. Noble, J., Bourassa, M.G., Petitclerc, R., et al. *Myocardial bridging and milking effect of the left anterior descending coronary artery: Normal variant or obstruction.* Am J Cardiol 1976, 37: 993-9.
50. Nakamura, M., Takeshita, A., Nose, Y. *Clinical characteristics associated with myocardial infarction, arrhythmias and sudden death in patients with vasospastic angina.* Circulation 1987, 75: 1110-7.
51. Torner, P., Brugada, P., Smeets, J., et al. *Ventricular fibrillation in the Wolff-Parkinson-White syndrome.* Eur Heart J 1991, 12: 144-50.
52. Della Bella, P., Brugada, P., Talajic, M., et al. *Atrial fibrillation in patients with an accessory pathway: Importance of the conduction properties of the accessory pathway.* J Am Coll Cardiol 1991, 17: 1352-6.

53. Moss, A.J., Schwartz, P.J., Crampton, R.S., et al. *The long QT syndrome: Prospective longitudinal study of 328 families.* Circulation 1991, 84: 1136-44.
54. Schwartz, P.J., Priori, S.G. *Clinical utility of QT interval monitoring.* In: Noninvasive Electrocardiology. Clinical Aspects of Holter Monitoring. A.J. Moss, S. Stern (Eds.). W.B. Saunders Company Ltd.: London 1996, 465-74.
55. Brugada, J., Brugada, R., Brugada, P. *Right bundle-branch block and ST-segment elevation in leads V1 through V3: A marker for sudden death in patients with demonstrable structural heart disease.* Circulation 1998, 97(5): 457-60.
56. Nademanee, K., Veerakul, G., Nimmannit, S., et al. *Arrhythmogenic marker for the sudden unexplained death syndrome in Thai men.* Circulation 1997, 96: 2595-600.
57. Corrado, D., Thiene, G., Nava, A., Rossi, L., Pennelli, N. *Sudden death in young competitive athletes: Clinicopathologic correlations in 22 cases.* Am J Med 1990, 89: 588-96.
58. Corrado, D., Basso, C., Thiene, G., et al. *Spectrum of clinicopathologic manifestations of arrhythmogenic right ventricular cardiomyopathy/dysplasia: A multicenter study.* J Am Coll Cardiol 1997, 30(6): 1512-20.
59. McKenna, W.J., Thiene, G., Nava, A., et al. *Diagnosis of arrhythmogenic right ventricular dysplasia/ cardiomyopathy. Task force of the working group myocardial and pericardial disease of the European Society of Cardiology and of the Scientific Council on Cardiomyopathies of the International Society and Federation of Cardiology.* Br Heart J 1994, 71: 215-8.
60. Bayés de Luna, A. Clinical Electrocardiography. A Textbook. 2nd Updated Edition. Futura Publishing Company, Inc.: Armonk, New York 1998.
61. Day, C.P., McComb, J.M., Campbell, R.W.F. *QT dispersion: An indication of arrhythmia risk in patients with long QT intervals.* Br Heart J, 1990, 63: 342-4.
62. Biffi, A., Ansalone, G., Verdile, L. *Ventricular arrhythmias and athlete's heart. Role of signal-averaged electrocardiography.* Eur Heart J 1996, 17: 557-63.
63. Marian A.J. *Sudden cardiac death in patients with hypertrophic cardiomyopathy: From bench to bedside with an emphasis on genetic markers.* Clin Cardiol 1995, 18: 189-98.
64. Vincent, G.M., Timothy, K.W., Leppert, M., Keating, M. *The spectrum of symptoms and QT intervals in carriers of the gene for the long-QT syndrome.* N Engl J Med 1992, 327: 846-52.
65. Rampazzo, A., Nava, A., Danieli, G.A., et al. *The gene for arrhythmogenic right ventricular cardiomyopathy maps to chromosome 14q23-q24.* Hum Mol Genet 1994, 3: 959-62.
66. Marian, A.J., Roberts, R. *Molecular genetic basis of hypertrophic cardiomyopathy: Genetic markers for sudden cardiac death.* J Cardiovasc Electrophysiol 1998, 9: 88-99.
67. Muller, J.E., Tofler, G.H., Stone, P.H. *Circadian variation and triggers of onset of acute cardiovascular disease.* Circulation 1989, 79: 733-43.
68. Mittleman, M.A., Maclure, M., Tofler, G.H., Sherwood, J.B., Godberg, R.J., Muller, J.E. *Triggering of acute myocardial infarction by heavy physical exertion. Protection against triggering by regular exertion.* N Engl J Med 1993, 329: 1677-83.
69. Willich, S.N., Lewis, M., Löwel, H., Arntz, H.R., Shubert, F., Schroder, F. *Physical exertion as a trigger of acute myocardial infarction. Triggers and mechanism of myocardial infarction group.* N Engl J Med 1993, 329: 1684-90.
70. Siscovick, D.S., Weiss, N.S., Fletcher, R.H., Lasky, T. *The incidence of primary cardiac arrest during vigorous exercise.* N Engl J Med 1984, 311: 874-7.
71. Lindinger, M.I. *Potassium regulation during exercise and recovery in humans: Implications for skeletal and cardiac muscle.* J Mol Cell Cardiol 1995, 27: 1011-22.
72. Stramba-Badiali, M., Guffanti, S., Porta, N., Frediani, M., Beria, G., Colnaghi, C. *QT interval prolongation and cardiac arrest during antibiotic therapy with spiramycin in a newborn infant.* Am Heart J 1993, 126: 740-2.
73. Woosley, R.L., Chen, Y., Freiman, J.P., Gillis, R.A. *Mechanism of the cardiotoxic action of terfenadine.* JAMA 1993, 269: 1532-6.
74. Wannamethee, G., Shaper, A.G. *Alcohol and sudden cardiac death.* Br Heart J 1992, 68: 443-8.
75. Nademanee, K. *Cardiovascular effects and toxicities of cocaine.* J Addict Dis 1992, 11: 71-82.
76. Maron, B.J., Poliac, LC., Kaplan, J.A., Mueller, F.O. *Blunt impact to the chest leading to sudden death from cardiac arrest during sports activities.* N Engl J Med 1995, 333(6): 337-42.
77. Link, M.S., Wang, P.J., Pandian, N.G., et al. *An experimental model of sudden death due to low-energy chest-wall impact (commotio cordis).* N Engl J Med 1998, 338: 1841-3.

CHAPTER 7

COMPETITIVE ATHLETES WITH ARRHYTHMIAS: CLASSIFICATION, EVALUATION AND TREATMENT

F. Furlanello[1], A. Bertoldi[2], F. Fernando[3] and A. Biffi[3]
[1]Istituto Scientifico H.S. Raffaele, Milan-Rome, Italy,
[2]Cardiology Department, Ospedale Civile S. Chiara, Trento, Italy and
[3]Istituto di Scienza dello Sport CONI, Rome, Italy

Background

Over the years great progress has been made in the treatment of arrhythmic patients, particularly in the understanding of the underlying electrophysiological mechanism and the utilization of nonpharmacological intervention therapies, such as the implantation of ventricular and atrial defibrillators or radiofrequency catheter ablation (1).

New frontiers are also opening up in the field of biology and molecular genetics with promising results in the areas of prevention, diagnosis and therapy, particularly concerning some specific inherited arrhythmogenic pathologies such as long QT syndrome, hypertrophic cardiomyopathy (HCM), arrhythmogenic right ventricular dysplasia (ARVD), progressive atrioventricular block, Brugada syndrome and atrial fibrillation (2-4).

Sports cardiology is also included in these, even though the results obtained at present are less exciting and leave large gaps in understanding the real significance of arrhythmias in athletes. The unpredictable onset and clinical context of these arrythmias limits a rational approach, especially with regard to the individuation of the risk that they can generate when combined with competitive sports activities.

However, immense efforts are also being made through contribution of cardiology in North America (5) to extend the practical benefits of modern arrhythmology to the athlete. Despite the lack of definitive information, valid conclusions have been reached regarding the risk of some types of arrhythmias during exercise, independent of the clinical substratum in which they occur (6), or the fact that they are a consequence or initial sign of certain cardiac pathologies that are known to cause sudden death (7). The latter are represented by various forms of cardiomyopathies, including: hypertrophic cardiomyopathy; dilated cardiomyopathy (DCM); ARVD; coronary heart disease (CHD) (atherosclerotic and congenital); myocarditis in its various phases (acute, healing, healed); valvular or congenital diseases such as mitral valve prolapse; aortic stenosis; primary alterations of the cardiac conduction system and primary arrhythmic disorders, such as congenital long QT syndrome in its various types (2); and "idiopathic" ventricular fibrillation including also the subgroups such as Brugada syndrome and polymorphic ventricular tachycardia with normal QT "short-coupled variant of torsade de pointes" (8).

89

A. Bayés de Luna et al. (eds.), Arrhythmias and Sudden Death in Athletes, 89–105.
© 2000 Kluwer Academic Publishers. Printed in the Netherlands.

However, many arrhythmias are benign and in athletes can coexist with normal physical performance without risk; they can be transitory, nonprogressive and induced or accentuated by modifications of the autonomic nervous system due to the sports activity.

In athletes with serious arrhythmias it is necessary to obtain the following data: evaluation of the clinical and prognostic significance of the identified arrhythmia in each individual athlete in relation to the specific sport activity in the short-, medium- and long-term; presence of an underlying arrhythmogenic heart disease or a primary arrhythmic disorder for which the arrhythmia acts as an expression, marker or consequence; immediate identification of a transient arrhythmogenic situation, such as infectious diseases, thyroid dysfunction, intake of illicit drugs, nutrition, metabolic disorders, etc. (9).

In subjects with arrhythmias classified as at-risk, borderline or dubious, it is necessary to implement a prolonged, comprehensive, clinical surveillance, if pharmacological and/or intervention treatment is also required (10) (Table 1).

Table 1. Competitive athletes with arrhythmias. The purpose of an arrhythmological study.

1.	To perform a detailed, individual diagnosis and prognosis for the suspected arrhythmias
2.	To search for any underlying heart disease or primary arrhythmic disorders
3.	To rule out any infectious, metabolic, electrolyte, toxic, etc. situations
4.	To classify the recognized arrhythmias concerning sports eligibility
5.	To make the final decisions concerning sports eligibility
6.	To implement a prolonged clinical surveillance and pharmacological and/or interventional treatment in dubious, borderline and high risk cases

Classification of Arrhythmias in the Competitive Athlete

The classification of cardiac arrhythmias is undergoing substantial modifications thanks to the data obtained from the new morphofunctional tridimensional acquisitions taken from intracardiac catheter ablation (11). This classification can also be useful for athletes; however, for a practical approach it is still useful to classify arrhythmias in competitive athletes who require evaluation of sports eligibility as "benign", "paraphysiological" and "pathological" (10) (Table 2). Immediate recognition of the nature of the arrhythmia is not always easy. At times it can be identified in an individual athlete after an extensive diagnostic protocol, which may also include an invasive diagnostic protocol, frequently completed with a close follow-up.

BENIGN ARRHYTHMIAS
Benign arrhythmias in an athlete are those arrhythmias which i) do not represent a risk factor for cardiac arrest; ii) do not induce hemodynamic consequences during athletic activity due to excessive bradycardia or tachycardia; and iii) are not markers of an underlying arrhythmogenic heart disease which in itself is enough to consider the athlete ineligible for competitive sport activities, such as arrhythmogenic right ventricular dysplasia, hypertrophic cardiomyopathy, dilated cardiomyopathy, coronary heart disease, congenital long QT syndrome, etc.

Table 2. Classification of competitive athletes with arrhythmias.

Benign	Compatible with sport eligibility
Paraphysiological	Due to prolonged athletic training
Pathological	Due to hemodynamic effects on the athletic performance and sports career
	Due to arrhythmogenic substratum: Structural heart disease or primary arrhythmic disorders
	At risk for cardiac arrest, sudden death

1 - Arrhythmias have to be considered benign only after a precise identification.
2 - Paraphysiological arrhythmias are "typical" of competitive athletes and compatible with sport eligibility.
3 - Athletes with transient pathological arrhythmias may have their sports eligibility restored (after radiofrequency catheter ablation, nonfatal commotio cordis, healed myocarditis, etc.).

Benign arrhythmias in athletes can also be considered those which are associated with an underlying heart disease such as mitral valve prolapse or Wolff-Parkinson-White (WPW) syndrome, in which an accurate arrhythmological study confirms that the anomaly is compatible with competitive sport activity. The solution is difficult in borderline cases, including: i) idiopathic repetitive ventricular tachycardia originating from the outflow tract of the pulmonary artery, a condition which is well tolerated in the absence of an underlying heart disease; ii) numerous ventricular ectopic beats (VEB) with sporadic couplets, which disappear under stress and with no apparent underlying heart disease; iii) frequent, complex, asymptomatic supraventricular ectopic beats (SVEB) in which it is fundamental to rule out silent ischemic heart disease, myocarditis, hyperthyroidism, intake of "arrhythmogenic" substances including illicit ones (*i.e.*, cocaine, amphetamines, etc); or iv) episodes of non-fast reentrant supraventricular tachycardia which the athlete apparently tolerates well with no repercussion on his/her athletic performance. Therefore, the classification of arrhythmia as benign in an athlete can at times be a difficult task both from a diagnostic and a prognostic point of view.

PARAPHYSIOLOGICAL ARRHYTHMIAS

The following characteristics of arrhythmias are common in athletes: arrhythmias usually disappear or are reduced with the cessation of training; they are a consequence of intense, prolonged and systematic training, especially if started at a young age (*e.g.*, in activities such as soccer, basketball, gymnastics, swimming, dancing, etc.); and they are also seen in athletes who compete under special conditions, including sports played under water or at a high altitude, and endurance sports such as long distance cycling, marathon running, cross country skiing, etc.

Paraphysiological arrhythmias are characterized by bradyarrhythmia, which is present at rest and disappears during exercise, and includes: sinus bradycardia, even marked (up to values of 25 bpm); sinus pauses (>2 sec); first degree and second degree intermittent Mobitz 1 atrioventricular (AV) blocks; "wandering" pacemaker; junctional and ventricular escape beats, leading to bradycardia and isorhythmic atriojunctional dissociation; and slow ventricular tachycardia (between 60 and 120 bpm). All these paraphysiological arrhythmias must disappear during exercise.

Problems of differential diagnosis occur with the "pathological bradyarrhythmias" when i) sinus or atrioventricular pauses are very prolonged (>3 sec) and they are not only intermittent but present at rest during the day; when the first degree AV block is very prolonged (>26 msec); and when the bradyarrhythmias are "atypical", e.g., second degree AV block unclearly Mobitz 1.

A difficult diagnostic problem usually requiring an electrophysiological endocavitary study with His bundle recording of the blockage site, which can be supra-Hisian (vagally mediated) or infra-Hisian, occurs in cases with Mobitz II appearance but with a unwidened QRS, a preexistent bundle-branch block, or when the block is induced during exercise despite being proximal (12) . Attention has to be paid to marked bradyarrhythmias in relation to the degree of training of an athlete when there is a family history of sudden death and symptoms such as fatigue, vertigo, light-headedness, syncope. Finally, these arrhythmias lead to the suspicion of pathological anomalies of the conduction system, which may be congenital or acquired, involve the sinoatrial node, the atrioventricular node and surrounding areas, the His bundle including its branches (13) .

In conclusion, paraphysiological bradyarrhythmias in athletes are highly prevalent in many types of competitive sports and are easily diagnosed due to the fact that they disappear during exercise and after a lapse in training; however, in a certain number of cases they require a thorough arrhythmological evaluation to rule out primary and secondary anomalies, whether congenital or acquired, of the cardiac conduction system.

PATHOLOGICAL ARRHYTHMIAS

Arrythmias are considered "pathological" when they are preclusive of sports eligibility, especially in the following cases:

1) When they are markers or the consequence of a silent arrhythmogenic heart disease or of a primary arrhythmic disorder such as arrhythmogenic right ventricular dysplasia (14-16); hypertrophic cardiomyopathy (17); coronary heart disease (congenital or atherosclerotic); dilated cardiomyopathy; myocarditis (acute, subacute or healed); risk of mitral valve prolapse; certain forms of valvular heart diseases (e.g., aortic stenosis); risk of WPW syndrome; congenital and acquired long QT syndrome; and pathological anomalies of the conduction system at different levels.

2) When they have hemodynamic consequences on the cardiovascular system and on athletic performance due to excessive tachycardia or bradycardia; frequent number of episodes and/or long duration; and abrupt onset and cessation. They can be divided into the following categories: i) arrhythmias which alone are not life threatening but which can interfere with the competitive athletic activity since they appear during or immediately after physical exercise (especially if they occur in sports with a high intrinsic risk, such as motor sports, underwater sports, alpine skiing, parachuting, etc.), such as paroxysmal atrial fibrillation and flutter (18), rapid reentry paroxysmal supraventricular tachycardia, marked bradyarrhythmia, sinus arrest or paroxysmal AV blocks, right or left idiopathic ventricular tachycardia; and ii) life-threatening arrhythmias capable of inducing symptoms, such as fainting, presyncope, syncope, cardiac arrest, and athletic activity related sudden death (Table 3), particularly rapid sustained ventricular tachycardia, torsade de pointes, ventricular fibrillation, rapid preexcited atrial fibrillation, and prolonged asystole due to paroxysmal sinus atrial block and AV block.

Table 3. Life-threatening arrhythmias in competitive athletes
causing severe symptoms, syncope, cardiac arrest and sudden death.

Bradyarrhythmias inducing prolonged asystole or polymorphic VT, torsades de pointes, VT/VF:
  Sinoatrial block
  Atrioventricular supra-infraHisian block

Supraventricular arrhythmias inducing rapid heart/rate/VT/VF:
  Atrial fibrillation with an underlying structural heart disease
  Atrial flutter with an underlying structural heart disease
  Wolff-Parkinson-White syndrome and rapid preexcited atrial fibrillation

Ventricular arrhythmias:
  In structural heart disease also in early phases
      DCM, HCM, ARVD, CAD, myocarditis, etc.
  From primary arrhythmic disorders
      Idiopathic VT/VF
      Short coupled variant of torsades de pointes with normal QT
      Brugada syndrome

Congenital long QT syndrome

VT= ventricular tachycardia; VF = ventricular fibrillation; DCM = dilated cardiomyopathy; HCM = hypertrophic cardiomyopathy; ARVD = arrhythmogenic right ventricular dysplasia; CAD = coronary artery disease; Brugada syndrome: right bundle-branch block, ST elevation in right precordial leads, clinical and/or induced VT/VF.

In certain cases a life-threatening arrhythmia can also be considered atrial flutter with a rapid AV conduction during exercise, mainly in the presence of an underlying structural heart disease (19). Belonging to this group of pathological arrhythmias are those forms which are at high risk of recurrence of cardiac arrest and sudden death and which are at the present time classified as idiopathic, or in which an underlying substratum has not been diagnosed, such as idiopathic ventricular fibrillation (20); polymorphic ventricular tachycardia ("short-coupled variant of torsades de pointes", without long QT) (8); and Brugada syndrome (21) involving ST elevation in the right precordial leads, right bundle-branch block, spontaneous and/or inducible ventricular tachycardia/fibrillation with high risk of sudden death. One must also keep in mind the possibility that a similar ECG finding in young subjects having experienced a sudden cardiac death can also be associated with a specific underlying cardiac anomaly such as ARVD (22).

"Commotio cordis" is a recognized cause of a form of difficult-to-manage cardiac arrest and sudden cardiac death, which occurs as consequence of a nonpenetrating precordial thoracic trauma caused by an abrupt blow (not extremely violent) usually caused by a baseball ball, hockey puck or softball ball. This usually occurs in young athletes in whom both *in vivo* and careful anatomopathological examinations frequently do not show any thoracic or cardiac damage (23). The arrhythmic mechanism is probably a ventricular fibrillation induced by a critical destabilization such as an R-on-T phenomenon. Cases of asystole have also been documented, as was found in one high ranking rugby player in our arrhythmic athletic population (24-26) who on violent impact with an opponent during competition had a subsequent asystolic cardiac arrest. The athlete recovered with no apparent problems thanks to the immediate intervention of the medical team present on field.

Management of the Arrhythmic Athlete

At the present time some guidelines are available, such as those established by the Bethesda Consensus Conference in 1994 (27), which are widely described in the monography (5) on sudden death in athletes. In Italy, we have cardiological guidelines such as the COCIS '95 (28) for the assessment of competitive sports eligibility, which is the result of different opinions originating from various cardiological and sports medicine associations, including the Italian Society of Cardiology (SIC), National Association of Hospital Cardiologists (ANMCO), Italian Society of Sports Cardiology (SIC Sport), National Association of Out of Hospital Cardiologists (ANCE) and the Italian Sports Medicine Federation (FMSI), in which a wide variety of options is given for the practical management of the athlete with suspected or documented arrhythmias.

Italian sports legislation requires a medical certificate for an athlete to be eligible to perform in his/her specific activity and imposes a thorough arrhythmological evaluation to assess the arrhythmic risk and eventual underlying heart disease and to exclude life-threatening arrhythmia that is incompatible with a career in sports. Clinical surveillance must be established and performed in at-risk cases (15,16,24-26).

The athlete with arrhythmias can undergo **three different levels** of evaluation (29, 30) as shown below.

The first level involves a check-up performed by a sports physician is necessary to be eligible to take part in a competitive sports activity. This includes a thorough personal and family history, a clinical exam with an ECG at rest and after a step test. Usually after this visit 3-4% of the athletes are considered ineligible, 60-86% of whom for cardiovascular problems and 25-37% for arrhythmic manifestations (31-33).

The second level includes a cardiological observation combined with all the necessary noninvasive diagnostic techniques (Table 4) as follows:

i) Family history with particular emphasis on cases of sudden cardiac death especially occurring at a young age; right ventricular arrhythmogenic dysplasia (34); hypertrophic cardiomyopathy; congenital long QT syndrome; Marfan's syndrome; mitral valve prolapse; WPW syndrome; congenital AV block (2); idiopathic ventricular fibrillation; and Brugada syndrome (21).

ii) Personal history focusing on symptoms, especially if they are related to exercise, such as palpitations, light-headedness, presyncope, syncope, precordial pain, dyspnea, and unjustifiable reduction in athletic performance. It must always be kept in mind that prodromal symptoms can be present up to even 60% of the cases in young athletes (<35 years) with severe arrhythmic events such as "on-field" cardiac arrest (24-26). Cases of hyperthermia, inflammatory-infective diseases, autoimmune, metabolic and endocrine disorders (*e.g.*, thyroid dysfunction), bronchial asthma, epilepsy, etc., use of potentially arrhythmogenic substances (especially in subjects with a particular predisposition) otherthan illicit drugs (9), such as β_2-adrenergic stimulants, erythromycin, pentamidine, psychotropic drugs, terfenadine, some types of organic phosphate insecticides, probucol, haloperidol, cocaine, etc. (35) should also be monitored.

Table 4. Competitive athletes with arrhythmias. Noninvasive (2nd level) investigation.

Family and personal history
Clinical visit
Resting and stress test ECG
Holter monitoring, also during intense physical activity
M and 2 Doppler color flow echocardiography
Stress echography, pharmacological and during exercise
Transesophageal echocardiography
Magnetic resonance imaging
Nuclear cardiology
Myocardial perfusion imaging
Radionuclide angiography
I 123 meta-iodobenzylguanidine scintigraphy
Signal averaged ECG time and frequency domain analysis
Uphead tilt-test
Transesophageal atrial pacing
Routine blood tests
Specific blood test (*i.e.,* for myocarditis)
Search for illicit substances
Genetic research

iii) Clinical check-up for xanthelasma, pectus excavatum, joint laxity, bone dysmorphism, eye defects (Marfan's syndrome) should be carried out as well as stetoacustic evaluation in different positions, Valsalva, etc. (mitral valve prolapse, obstructive hypertrophic cardiomyopathy, bicuspid aortic valve, etc.)

iv) Resting ECG should be carried out to monitor rhythm and heart rate, P-wave, atrioventricular or intraventricular conduction defects, long QT and its and spatial "dispersion", ventricular repolarization defects such as ST elevation-depression, and negative T-waves, particularly the right precordial leads, *e.g.*, as in right ventricular arrhythmogenic dysplasia (14-16, 34) and Brugada syndrome (21, 22) or more diffused as in hypertrophic cardiomyopathy, etc.

In athletes with WPW syndrome and in those with ventricular ectopic beats and/or VT it is possible to establish the spatial activation of the arrhythmia, *e.g.*, a right or left posterior septal accessory pathway localization for WPW syndrome, pulmonary outflow origin or left posterior septal origin of ventricular ectopic beats, VTs, etc.

v) Since athletes are being evaluated, a maximal stress test is necessary with continuous monitoring of the ECG to analyze the induction, aggravation, deterioration or reduction of the arrhythmia, if it is a bradycardia or tachyarrhythmia, and also to identify alterations in ventricular repolarization (Table 5).

A 12 lead stress test is an excellent method to identify the spatial origin of the ventricular arrhythmia (right, left, septal, apex, outflow tract and duration, and spatial dispersion of QT, etc.). The sophisticated stress test systems now available will in the future be a useful tool in the risk stratification of the arrhythmic athlete. These include highfrequency analysis (during stress-test or pacing) of micro T-wave alternans, which is a noninvasive diagnostic technique for arrhythmic electrical vulnerability and is apparently highly

Table 5. Competitive athletes with arrhythmias. The role of ECG ambulatory monitoring.

The introduction of ECG ambulatory monitoring in sports cardiology (1974) had a tremendous impact totally overtaking the previous use of ECG telemetry for:
Search for a normality standard in the athletic population
Paraphysiological arrhythmic manifestations induced by training (bradyarrhythmias, SA-AV block), sometimes very impressive
High prevalence of ectopic beats in "normal" athletes
Possible identification of life-threatening arrhythmias in asymptomatic athletes, including elite athletes
The Holter monitoring at rest and during exercise became mandatory in the diagnosis and prognosis of the arrhythmic athlete

predictive in some cases of arrhythmogenic cardiopathy, such as long QT syndrome, coronary artery disease, hypertrophic and dilated cardiomyopathy, mitral valve prolapse, electrolyte-metabolic disorders and drug effects (36-38).

vi) Holter monitoring (Table 6) is considered a fundamental diagnostic technique in the evaluation of the arrhythmic athlete (39-42) and must include moments of intense physical activity and when possible, recorded while the athlete is performing his or her specific activity. A good Holter monitoring gives us useful information in approximately 50% of the studied cases in terms of sports eligibility (43).

Table 6. Competitive athletes with arrhythmias. Clinical role of ECG ambulatory monitoring.

1) Current indication
Any arrhythmic environmental events: number, percentage, type, day/night distribution (variability of the ECG parameters included), symptoms and patient's activity correlation
Transient symptomatic arrhythmic event:
Long term (day, weeks) with no implantable ECG recorder

2) Special applications (still to be established in athletes)
Long-term analysis of QT intervals:
(QT interval-heart rate relation, circadian patterns of QT duration)
i.e., in patients with congenital long QT syndrome of different types (1, 2, 3)
With acquired long QT (*i.e.,* for different drugs)
Heart rate variability both in time and frequency domain in short- and long-term analysis
Risk stratification of cardiac death
(Post MI patients, DCM, CHF, etc.)
Initiating mechanisms of VT, VF
(*i.e.,* in patients with ICD) or AF

See table 3 for abbreviations

New possibilities have also emerged for risk stratification with the long-term QT interval analysis and heart rate variability (according to time and frequency domain in short- and long-term analysis) (Table 7) even if there are as yet no conclusive studies concerning athletes.

vii) M and 2D Doppler color flow echocardiography is an invaluable diagnostic technique for the morphological evaluation of the heart in the arrhythmic athlete with particular regard to dilated and hypertrophic cardiomyopathy, valvular, ischemic, myocarditis

Table 7. Competitive athletes with arrhythmias.
Transesophageal atrial pacing at rest and during exercise.

Indications
All inducible recurrent supraventricular tachycardias
Atrioventricular nodal reentry tachycardia
Atrioventricular reentry tachycardia of overt or concealed and preexcited atrial fibrillation in
Wolff-Parkinson White syndrome (risk stratification)
Atrial fibrillation and flutter
Idiopathic left "verapamil-like" ventricular tachycardia
Screening of sinus node and atrioventricular bradyarrhythmias

and ARVD. In expert hands it can also allow for the detection of an anomalous origin and course of the coronary arteries (44). It can also be implemented with stress echography, pharmacologically (which is less used in athletes) and during exercise (silent ischemic heart disease). The latter is a "physiological" technique with detailed Italian experiments (45, 46). Transesophageal echocardiography (pathologies of the aorta, mitral, tricuspid, atrial septal defect, intraatrial formations, ARVD, etc.) can also be used.

viii) Magnetic resonance imaging (MRI) is a fundamental diagnostic technique for detecting an underlying organic substrate, particularly in ARVD and those arrhythmias with right ventricular origin (*e.g.*, outflow tract of the pulmonary artery) (47-50), and also in other cases such as myocarditis and hypertrophic cardiomyopathy. Recently an important role in the noninvasive diagnostic evaluation of ARVD and silent coronary cardiopathy has been obtained with "electron beam computed tomography imaging" capable of giving functional information and also tissue information, (coronary calcifications, fatty infiltration), considered superior to NMR (51, 52).

ix) For nuclear cardiology the most useful radioisotopic diagnostic techniques in the arrhythmic athlete are myocardial perfusion imaging at rest and during stress to identify a silent coronary artery disease (52); radionuclide angiography at rest and during stress that allows for a good evaluation of the ejection fraction, and is used for coronary artery disease, myocarditis, dilated cardiomyopathy and ARVD (53); MIBG (I 123 meta-iodobenzylguanidine) scintigraphy for the evaluation of the cardiac neuroadrenergic function, being particularly useful in the diagnosis of early stage of ARVD, the extension of this disease to the left ventricle (54-55) and for identification of some silent cardiomyopathy.

x) Signal averaged ECG time and frequency domain (spectral turbulence technique) is used in the early diagnosis of the arrhythmogenic substrate and in risk stratification in athletes with arrhythmias, which are usually ventricular, and particularly in the subclinical stage (56-59). It is also particularly used in ARVD, coronary artery disease, hypertrophic cardiomyopathy, mitral valve prolapse, etc. It is a noninvasive diagnostic technique which has been widely adopted in sports arrhythmology in Italy, especially in the time domain, with major limitations due to the presence of false positives and to the fact that the population usually has a low incidence of the disease investigated.

xi) Uphead tilt-test is conducted at rest and after a pharmacological test (*i.e.*, sublingual nitrates) (60) and is a very important technique in the screening of subjects with episodes of vasovagal, vasodepressive or cardioinhibitory syncope, which are not rare in trained athletes (61).

xii) Transesophageal atrial pacing (TAP) (Table 7) at rest and during exercise (bicycle ergometer test) is a very important test for all the "inducible" supraventricular tachycardias, particularly for reentrant atrioventricular tachycardia (AVRT) in WPW syndrome, atrioventricular node reentrant tachycardia (NAVRT), and to evaluate the risk factors in athletes with WPW syndrome, even if they are asymptomatic (62-64), as well as in paroxysmal atrial flutter and fibrillation, and in some forms of "verapamil-like" idiopathic ventricular tachycardias. It is also useful in the screening of sinus and atrioventricular bradyarrhythmias.

xiii) Blood tests include routine blood tests such as thyroid function tests (FT3, FT4 and thyroid-stimulating hormone), liver and kidney function tests, and markers for inflammation and rheumatic diseases; specific tests such as a search for viral, bacterial, mycotic, parasitic, spirochetal, rickettsial, drug-related and autoimmune related agents of myocarditis (65); and tests to detect illicit substances that can cause arrhythmias in athletes, such as amphetamines, anabolic steroids, corticosteroids, cocaine, etc. With regard to substances such as erythropoietin, it is as yet only possible to conduct an indirect haematocrit evaluation.

Genetic testing can also be carried out as some arrhythmic pathologies have a genetic cause, such as the long QT syndrome (in all its various subtypes), hypertrophic cardiomyopathy, ARVD, WPW syndrome, progressive AV block, idiopathic ventricular fibrillation including the Brugada syndrome, for which it would be useful to obtain molecular genetic data on short notice for diagnostic purposes (initial forms, dubious, silent) and prognosis. Genetic typing is already available for congenital long QT syndrome, hypertrophic cardiomyopathy and Brugada syndrome. Unfortunately, the laboratories that conduct these exams are few, the execution time for the tests are long and the results are often uncertain. For a rational use of the present resources these analyses (blood sampling in every family member with overt or suspected pathologies) are preferably dedicated to large groups where the possibility of obtaining useful data is easier to predict (2).

The second level arrhythmological tests have in common only the fact that they can be performed at an outpatient laboratory level. They include basic investigations such as stress testing, echocardiography, Holter monitoring (25) and also more complex ones that require a highly specialized laboratory.

Finally, **the third level** of invasive diagnostic techniques are conducted in a limited number of arrhythmic competitive athletes but sometimes are indispensable for the correct diagnosis and eventual therapeutic approach. The athlete must be informed thoroughly of all the risks and benefits of the invasive procedures.

Invasive Diagnostic Techniques to Identify and Evaluate the Underlying Heart Disease

Cardiac catheterization, contrast ventriculography and angiography and coronary arteriography can be conducted when necessary for congenital coronary disease or atherosclerosis, acquired or congenital valvular disease, and primary or secondary cardiomyopathy including ARVD.

Endomyocardial biopsy can be carried out particularly to diagnose myocarditis (65) (excluding usually the acute forms), ARVD (66) and other forms of cardiomyopathy if not otherwise diagnosed.

Invasive Arrhythmologic Investigation

Invasive arrhythmologic investigation involves an in-depth diagnosis including techniques such as radiofrequency catheter ablation and implantable cardioverter defibrillator (ICD).

Endocavitary electrophysiological study can be conducted for paroxysmal atrial fibrilloflutter, persistent or recurring tachycardia (reentry or ectopic focus) which is atrial, nodal, right or left ventricular (idiopathic or organic), when necessary for diagnostic, prognostic and therapeutic approach; WPW and other ventricular preexcitations (*i.e.*, Mahaim) for diagnosis and risk stratification; severe symptoms, presyncope, syncope of possible arrhythmic origin, and in subjects recovered for cardiac arrest; the diagnosis of a wide complex tachycardia (aberration of the intraventricular conduction *vs.* ventricular tachycardia); electrical exitoconduction defects which are sinoatrial, AV, intraventricular and paraphysiological in the athlete (see above); risk stratification in athletes with complex ventricular ectopic beats, unsustained and sustained VT, especially when they coexist with high risk factors (structural heart disease, positive late ventricular potentials, etc.); any indication for radiofrequeny catheter ablation prior to thorough clinical indication screening, preferably combining the procedure during the same electrophysiological evaluation to avoid discomfort for the subject (Table 8); and electropharmacological testing particularly for VT as an indication for ICD implantation in high-risk patients.

Table 8. Competitive athletes with arrhythmias. Radiofrequency catheter ablation.

Indications
All supraventricular reentry and focal tachycardias:
Recurrent or incessant, need of antiarrythmic drug treatment
Not compatible with sports eligibility
Wolff-Parkinson-white syndrome symptomatic and/or at risk
Atrial flutter
Individual cases of continuously recurrent atrial fibrillation (focal elision or linear lesions) of right and/or left atrium, particularly with tridimensional nonfluoroscopic approach
Idiopathic, right or left ventricular tachycardia
Management of VT in structural heart disease (ARVD, DCM, CAD, etc.)

For abbreviations see Table 3.

Pacemaker implantation, preferably rate responsive and by chamber (*i.e.*, DDDR) (even atrial "multisites") can be used in symptomatic overt sick sinus syndrome, and in third degree AV block, congenital supra-Hisan or acquired supra-infraHisan (frequently paroxysmal and symptomatic).

Mono or dual chamber ICD implantation in malignant ventricular arrhythmias can be used in (Table 9) structural heart disease (especially if progressive, *i.e.*, arrhythmogenic right ventricular dysplasia, dilated and hypertrophic cardiomyopathy, postmyocardial infarction cardiomyopathy).

Table 9. Competitive athletes with arrhythmias. With ICD implantation.

Indications
Malignant ventricular arrhythmias: recurrent, refractory, unstable VT, torsade de pointes, polymorphic VT, VF, cardiac arrest with CPR (not due to transient causes)
a) From structural heart disease, particularly if progressive: ARVD, DCM, HCM, CAD, etc.

b) From primary arrhythmic disorders at high risk of recurrences, cardiac arrest, sudden death:
   Idiopathic VT/VF
   Brugada syndrome
   Congenital long QT, presented with cardiac arrest or with syncope refractory to betablockers and left
   stellectomy

For abbreviations see Table 3

Primary arrhythmic disorders, with a high risk of recurrences, cardiac arrest, sudden death, include: idiopathic ventricular tachycardia/fibrillation, Brugada syndrome and congenital long QT (presented with cardiac arrest).

Personal Experiences in the Treatment of Arrhythmic Young Competitive Elite Athletes

From 1974 to January 1999, 1,952 young competitive athletes (with previous eligibility to take part in competitive sport activities) were included in an individualized arrhythmological study based on a codified clinical and instrumental protocol (10, 15, 16, 18, 24-26, 29, 40, 41, 67, 68). Subjects included 1,637 males and 315 females with a mean age of 21.4 years who all had arrhythmias that endangered their sports career (Table 10).

Table 10. Competitive athletes with arrhythmias.
Summary of the population studied from 1974 to January 1999.

Athletes	Number	Male	Female	Average age (years)	Follow-up (months) min-max	Number with sudden death	Number with cardiac arrest
All athletes	1952	1637	315	21.4	3-123	21 (1.1%)	31 (1.6%)
Elite athletes	161	134	27	27	3-109	3 (1.9%)	4 (2.5%)

Twenty-one athletes experienced sudden cardiac death; this occurred as the first symptom in seven (33.3%), three of which were due to atherosclerotic coronary artery disease and four to myocarditis, and in 14 during the follow-up period (72.2%). Thirty-one athletes were studied after a documented cardiac arrest and resuscitation by CPR. Twenty-nine cases were related to exercise and two occurred at rest (one had WPW and another dilated cardiomyopathy). Cardiac arrest was due to ventricular tachycardia/ventricular fibrillation in 28 (90%), commotio cordis with asystole in one and third degree paroxysmal AV block in two.

A total of 161 out of 1,952 subjects (134 males and 25 females) with an average age 25 years were elite athletes and included Italian, European, World and Olympic Champions. Of these 161 athletes, 68 (42.2%) had an underlying cardiac abnormality (69) (Table 11) as follows: arrhythmogenic right ventricular dysplasia in 12 (7.5%); mitral valve prolapse in 27 (16.6%); dilated cardiomyopathy in three (1.9%), one with sudden death; hypertrophic cardiomyopathy in one (0.6%); WPW syndrome in 15 (9.3%), one being an alpine skier who was asymptomatic but had been identified at risk, and who had cardiac arrest (at night) as the first symptom; severe mitral incontinence in one (0.6%); aortic valve disease in three (1.9%); myocarditis in four (2.5%); atherosclerotic coronary artery disease one (0.6%), with sudden death at night as first symptom; and unknown cardiomyopathy in one (0.6%) with sudden death, during follow-up.

Table 11. Cardiac abnormalities in 161 elite athletes with arrhythmias.

Disease	Total athletes	% of total elite athletes	Sudden death	Cardiac arrest
Arrhythmogenic right ventricular dysplasia	12	7.5		1
Mitral valve prolapse	27	16.7		
Wolff-Parkinson-White syndrome	15	9.3		1
Dilated cardiomyopathy	3	1.9	1	1
Hypertrophic cardiomyopathy	1	0.6		1
Mitral regurgitation (severe)	1	0.6		
Aortic valvular disease	3	1.9		
Myocarditis	4	2.5		
Coronary artery disease	1	0.6	1	
Unknown cardiomyopathy	1	0.6	1	
Total	68	42.2	3	4

Of these 161 athletes, 73 (45.4%) were considered ineligible to take part in competitive sport activities, 18 (24.6%) were under antiarrhythmic treatment, four (2.5%) had previously documented cardiac arrest, three were affected on field (one rugby player with asystolic commotio cordis during a game, one (ARVD) during an uphill cycling competition, one during a soccer practice), at rest at night in one (WPW); 11 had arrhythmic nonfatal syncope including two with asystolic vasovagal syndrome. One, a rugby player at a very high international level, succumbed to sudden death at night, as a first symptom; atherosclerotic obstructive coronary artery disease was documented at pathological examination.

During the follow-up period (minimum 3, maximum 109 months) the following occurred: two ex-elite athletes (with ARVD) required ICD implantation for refractory

fast VT and high risk of sudden death; two experienced sudden death during unautho-
rized sport activity (both had been considered ineligible to compete due to a high arrhythmic risk); six elite athletes, with at-risk WPW (including the downhill skier with cardiac
arrest) had successful radiofrequency catheter ablation (RFCA) of the accessory pathway; two with refractory recurrent atrial fibrillation/flutter had successful atrial RFCA
using a tridimensional nonfluoroscopic approach.

Conclusions

This study shows and confirms that competitive and even elite athletes can have arrhythmic manifestations, including severe ones, which appear as markers or as a consequence
of underlying heart disease or primary arrhythmias which had previously not been diagnosed or had not been considered important. In these subjects, a systematic arrhythmological approach which is clinical and instrumental, especially at the second and third
level and includes noninvasive and invasive diagnostic techniques, allows us to differentiate at-risk forms which are incompatible with sports activity from those which allow,
under clinical surveillance, the continued participate in competitive sport activities.

In at-risk cases, a combination of restrictive measures and therapeutic ones, whether
pharmacological or interventional, including RFCA and ICD implantation, together with
a close follow-up are mandatory.

References

1. Farrè, J., Moro, C. (Eds). Ten Years of Radiofrequency Catheter Ablation. Futura Publishing Co, Inc.:
    Armonk, NY, 1998.
2. Priori, S., Napolitano, C. *Molecular diagnosis of inherited cardiac diseases: Impact on clinical practice.*
    G Ital Cardiol 1998, 28 (Suppl. 1): 273-8.
3. El-Sherif, N. *Advances in cardiac arrhythmias. From molecular biology to clinical management.* G Ital
    Cardiol 1998, 28 (Suppl. 1): 270-3.
4. Valente, M., Calabrese, F., Basso, C., Angelini, A., Thiene, G. *Apoptosis, cardiomyopathies and arrhyth-
    mias.* G Ital Cardiol 1998, 28 (Suppl. 1): 278-81.
5. Estes, N.A.M., Salem, D.N., Wang, P.J. (Eds.). Sudden Cardiac Death in the Athlete. Futura Publishing
    Co. Inc.: Armonk 1998.
6. Zipes, D.P. *Specific arrhythmias: Diagnosis and treatment.* In: Heart disease: A Textbook of
    Cardiovascular Medicine 5th Ed. Braunwald E. (Ed.). Saunders: Philadelphia 1997: 640-704.
7. Maron, B.J., Shirani, J., Poliac, L.C. et al. *Sudden death in young competitive athletes: Clinical, demo-
    graphic and pathological profiles.* JAMA 1996, 276: 199-204.
8. Jordaens, L., Tavernier, R., Kazmierczak, J., Dimmer, C. *Ventricular arrhythmias in apparently health
    subjects.* PACE 1997, 20 (Part III): 2692-8.
9. Kloner, R. *Illicit drug use in the athlete as a contributor to cardiac events.* In: Sudden Cardiac Death in
    the Athlete. Estes, N.A.M., Salem, D.N., Wang, P.J. (Eds). Futura Publishing Co., Inc.: Armonk 1998:
    441-51.
10. Furlanello, F., Bertoldi, A., Bettini, R., Dallago, M., Vergara, G.I. *Life threatening tachyarrhythmias in
    athletes.* PACE 1992, 15: 1403-12.
11. Cosio, F., Anderson, R., Kuch, K., on behalf of the Cardiac Nomenclature Study Group of the Working
    Group of Arrhythmias of the European Society of Cardiology. *New Classification of Cardiac Arrhythmias.*

To understand atrial arrhythmias, we need to make nomenclature match anatomy! G Ital Cardiol 1998, 28 (Suppl. 1): 411-15.

12. Sumiyoshi, M., Nakata, Y., Yasuda, M. *Clinical and electrophysiologic features of exercise-induced atrioventricular block.* Am Heart J 1996, 132: 1277.

13. Bharati, S. *The cardiac conduction system in sudden death in athletes.* In: Sudden Cardiac Death in the Athlete. Estes, N.A.M., Salem, D.N., Wang, P.J. (Eds.). Futura Publishing Co., Inc.: Armonk, 1998: 483-514.

14. Nava, A., Rossi, L., Thiene, G. (Eds.). Arrhythmogenic Right Ventricular Cardiomyopathy/Dysplasia. Elsevier Science B.V.: Amsterdam 1997.

15. Furlanello F., Bertoldi A., Dallago M. et al. *Cardiac arrest and sudden death in competitive athletes with arrhythmogenic right ventricular dysplasia.* PACE 1998, 21 (Part II): 331-5.

16. Furlanello, F., Bertoldi, A., Bettini, R., Durante, GB., Vergara, G. *The disease in competitive athletes.* In: Arrhythmogenic Right Ventricular Cardiomyopathy/Dysplasia. Nava, A., Rossi, L., Thiene, G. (Eds.). Elsevier Science B.V.: Amsterdam 1997: 477-87.

17. Maron, B.J. *Hypertrophic cardiomyopathy as a cause of sudden death in the young competitive athlete in sudden death in young competitive athletes: Clinical, demographic and pathological profiles.* JAMA 1996, 16: 301-17.

18. Furlanello, F., Bertoldi A., Dallago M. et al. *Atrial fibrillation in elite athletes.* J Cardiovasc Electrophysiol 1998, 9 (Suppl.): 563-8.

19. Epstein, A.E., Mile, W.M., Benditt, D.G. *Personal and public safety issues related to arrhythmias that may affect consciousness: Implications for regulation and physician recommendations.* Circulation 1996, 94: 1147-66.

20. Priori, S., Paganini, V. *Idiopathic ventricular fibrillation. Epidemiology pathophysiology, primary prevention, immediate evaluation and management, long-term evaluation and management, experimental and theoretical developments.* Cardiac Electrophysiol Rev 1997, 1: 244-7.

21. Brugada, J., Brugada, P., Brugada, R. *Clinical and electrocardiographic patterns in patients with idiopathic ventricular fibrillation.* In: Ten Years of Radiofrequency Catheter Ablation. Farrè J., Moro C (Eds.). Futura Publishing Co. Inc.: Armonk 1998: 219-31.

22. Corrado, D., Basso, C., Buja, G., Nava, A., Thiene, G. *Right bundle branch block, right precordial ST segment elevation and sudden death in the young.* G Ital Cardiol 1998, (Suppl. 1): 566-8.

23. Link, M., Maron, B., Estes, M. *Commotio cordis.* In: Sudden Cardiac Death in the Athlete. Estes, N.A.M., Salem, D.N., Wang, P.J. (Eds.). Futura Publishing Co. Inc.: Armonk 1998: 515-28.

24. Bertoldi, A., Furlanello, F., Fernando, F. et al. *Young competitive athletes resuscitated from cardiac arrest on field: What have we learned and what can be done?* New Trends Arrhyth 1996, 1-4: 20-30.

25. Furlanello, F., Bertoldi, A., Dallago, M. et al. *Aborted sudden death in competitive athletes.* Prog Clin Pacing 1994, 51: 733-41.

26. Furlanello, F., Bertoldi, A., Fernando, F., Dallago, M., Inama, G., Vergara, G. *Estudio cardioaritmologico de jovenes atletas resuscitados de una muerte subita en el campo de juego.* Ed Lat Electrocard 1996, 2: 25-37.

27. Maron, B.J., Mitchell, J. *26th Bethesda Conference. Recommendations for determining eligibility for competition in athletes with cardiovascular abnormalities.* J Am Coll Cardiol 1994, 24: 848-99.

28. Comitato Organizzativo Cardiologico per l'idoneità allo Sport (COCIS). *Protocolli cardiologici per il giudizio di idoneità allo sport agonistico 1995.* G Ital Cardiol 1996, 26: 949-83.

29. Bertoldi, A., Furlanello, F., Fernando, F et al. *Cardioarrhythmologic evaluation of symptoms and arrhythmic manifestations in 110 top level consecutive professional athletes.* New Trends Arrhyth 1993, 9: 199-209.

30. Furlanello, F., Bertoldi, A., Fernando, F. *Current criteria for evaluation of athletes with arrhythmias.* In: Advances in Sports Cardiology. Pelliccia, A., Caselli, G., Bellotti, P. (Eds.). Springer-Verlag Italia: Milan 1997: 67-72.

31. Morandi, G., Schiavon, M. Epidemiologia delle Cause Cardiologiche di Inidoneità. Atti del VII Congresso Nazionale SIC. Sport. (Trento, 20-22 Sept. 1995), 153.

32. Frizzera, S., Bertoli, P., Resnyak, S. Cause di non Idoneità Cardiologiche: Rivalutazione Critica Dopo 12 Anni di Attività. Atti del VII Congresso Nazionale SIC. Sport, (Trento, 20-22 Sept. 1995), 154.

33. Fiorella, P.L., Cavallari, F., Bargossi, A.M. Le Causali Cardiologiche di Non Idoneità All'Attività Agonistica: Analisi del Fenomeno nella Regione Emilia Romagna. Atti del VII Congresso Nazionale SIC. Sport. (Trento, 20-22 Sept. 1995), 151-2.

34. Nava, A., Bauce, B., Villanova, C. et al. *Arrhythmogenic right ventricular cardiomyopathy: A report of 162 familial cases.* G Ital Cardiol 1998, 28 (Suppl. 1): 492-6.

35. Myerburg, R.J., Mitrani, R., Interian, A., Castellanos, A. *Identification of risk of cardiac arrest and sudden cardiac death in athletes.* In: Estes, N.A.M., Salem, D., Wang, P. Sudden Cardiac Death in the Athlete. Futura Publishing Co. Inc.: Armonk 1998, 25-55.

36. Corrado, D., Basso, C., Thiene, G. *Pathologic findings in victims of sports-related sudden cardiac death.* New Trends Arrhyth 1995, 11: 30-32.

37. Estes, N.A.M., Zipes, D.P., El-Sherif, N. et al. *Electrical alternans during rest and exercise as predictors of vulnerability to ventricular arrhythmias.* J Am Coll Cardio 1995, Feb.: 1027-39.

38. Armoundas, A.A., Rosenbaum, D.S., Ruskin, J.N., Garan, H., Cohen, R.J. *Electrophysiologic testing, electrical alternans and signal averaged eletrocardiography as predictors of arrhythmias-free survival.* J Am Cardio 1995, Feb.: 96-26.

39. Furlanello, F., Bertoldi, A., Dallago, M. et al. *Evaluation of cardiac arrhythmias in athletes.* J Ambul Monit 1991, 5: 285-97.

40. Furlanello, F., Bertoldi, A., Dallago, M. et al. *Evaluacion cardioarritmologica del atleta.* In: Cardiologia Deportiva. Bayes de Luna, A., Furlanello, F., Maron, B.J., Serra Grima, J.R. (Eds.). Doyma Libros: Barcelona 1994, 172-81.

41. Furlanello, F., Bettini, R., Bertoldi, A et al. *Competitive sports and cardiac arrhythmias.* In: Luderitz B., Saksena S. (Eds.). Interventional Electrophysiology. Futura Publishing: Mount Kisco., 1991: 41-7.

42. Furlanello, F., Bettini, R., Resina, A. *Mondiali di calcio 1990: 5 anni di sorveglianza aritmologica in calciatori della Nazionale Italiana.* In: Heart Surgery. D'Alessandro, L.C. (Ed.). CESI: Roma 1989, 631-4.

43. Kluge, P., Rose, E., Meyer, C. et al. *QT cynamics from holter recordings: A comparison of two averaging methods.* ANE 1998, 3(3): 232-6.

44. Zeppilli, P., Santini, C. *L'ecocardiogramma nell'atleta.* In: Cardiologia dello Sport. Zeppilli, P. (Ed.). CESI: Rome 1995: 197-242.

45. Penco, M. E*cocardiografia da sforzo.* In: Cardiologia dello Sport. Zeppilli, P. (Ed.). CESI: Roma 1995: 243-9.

46. Dagianti, A., Fedele, F., Penco, M. *Il Cardiologo dello Sport tra tecnologia e clinica nella diagnostica di ischemia miocardica.* Med. Sport 1993, 323-31.

47. Durante, G., Recla, M., Accardi, R. et al. Arrhythmogenic Right Ventricular Dysplasia (ARVD): Evaluation by Nuclear Magnetic Resonance. Proc 1st Int Symp on ARVD/C (Paris, June 16-18 1996) 11/39.

48. Penco, M., Di Cesare, E., Aurigemma, G. et al. *Arrhythmogenic right ventricular dysplasia: Which diagnostic role for magnetic resonance imaging?* G Ital Cardiol 1998, 28 (Suppl. 1): 475-81.

49. Molinari, G., Sardaneli., F., Gaita, F. et al. *Right ventricular dysplasia as a generalized cardiomyopathy? Findings on magnetic resonance imaging.* Eur Heart J 1995, 16: 1619-24.

50. Wichter, T., Lentschig, M.G., Reimer, P., Borggrefe, M., Breithard, G. *Magnetic resonance imaging.* In: Arrhythmogenic Right Ventricular Cardiomyopathy/Dysplasia. Nava, A., Rossi, L., Thiene, G. (Eds.). Elsevier Science B.V.: Amsterdam 1997, 269-84.

51. Tada, H., Shimizu, W., Ohe, T. et al. *Usefulness of electron-beam computed tomography in arrhythmogenic right ventricular dysplasia: Relationship to electrophysiological abnormalities and left ventricular involvement.* Circulation 1996, 94: 437-44.

52. Corrodi, J.G., Udelson, E.J. *Noninvasive imaging techniques to assess cardiac disease in the athlete.* In: Sudden Cardiac Death in the Athlete. Estes, N.A.M., Salem, D.N., Wang, P.J. (Eds) Futura Publishing Co. Inc.: Armonk 1998, 159-87.

53. Le Guludec, D., Slama, M., Faraggi, M. et al. *Radionuclide angiography.* In: Arrhythmogenic Right Ventricular Cardiomyopathy/Dysplasia. Nava, A., Rossi, L., Thiene, G. (Eds.). Elsevier Science B.V.: Amsterdam 1997, 285-97.

54. Bettini, R., Camerani, M., Severi, S., Furlanello, F. *MIBG scintigraphy in sportsmen.* In: Arrhythmogenic Right Ventricular Cardiomyopathy/Dysplasia. Nava, A., Rossi, L., Thiene, G. Elsevier Science B.V.: Amsterdam 1997, 463-76.

55. Witchter, T., Hindricks, G., Lerch, H. et al. *Regional myocardial sympathetic dysinnervation in arrhythmogenic right ventricular cardiomyopathy. An analysis using 123i-meta-iodebenzylguanidine scintigraphy.* Circulation 1994,89:667-83.
56. Biffi, A., Verdile, L., Caselli, G., et al. *Ventricular arrhythmias in athletes: Markers of subclinical heart disease.* G Ital Cardiol 1998, 28 (Suppl. 1): 519-21.
57. Bettini, R., Bonato, P., Furlanello, F. *Prevalence of late potentials in normal and arrhythmic athletes.* In: International Symposium on Progress in Clinical Pacing. Santini, M. (Ed.). Futura Media Service: Armonk 1994, 707.
58. Leclercq, J.F., Coumel, P. *Changes in surface ECG and signal-averaged ECG with time right ventricular dysplasia. Evidence for an evolving disease.* G Ital Cardiol 1998, 28 (Suppl. 1), 1998: 488-92.
59. Folino, F., Dal Corso, L., Oselladore, Luca., Nava, A. *Signal-averaged electrocardiogram.* In: Arrhythmogenic Right Ventricular Cardiomyopathy/Dysplasia. Nava A., Rossi L., Thiene G. (Eds.). Elsevier Science B.V.: Amsterdam 1997, 210-23.
60. Brignole, M., Menozzi, C., Gianfranchi, L. et al. *Carotid sinus massage, eyeball compression and head-up tilt test in patients with syncope of uncertain origin and in healthy control subjects.* Am Heart J 1991, 122: 1644.
61. Tortorella, G., Tomasi, C., Manari, A., Menozzi, C., Guiducci, U. *Syncope in middle-aged endurance athletes.* G Ital Cardiol 1998, 28 (Suppl. 1): 517.
62. Furlanello, F., Bertoldi, A., Fernando, F. *Progressi nell'approccio cardioaritmologico dell'atleta.* In: Convegno Nazionale - Firenze Aritmie. Disertori M., Marconi P. (Eds.). CSS: Florence 1997, 49-58.
63. Vergara, G., Furlanello, F., Disertori, M. et al. *Induction of supraventricular tachyarrhytmia at rest and during exercise with transesophageal atrial pacing in the electrophysiological evaluation of asymptomatic athletes with WPW syndrome.* Eur Heart J 1988, 9: 1119-26.
64. Furlanello, F., Bertoldi, A., Vergara, G. et al. *Cardiac Preexitation: What one should do in the selection and in the follow-up of an athlete.* Int J Sports Cardiol 1992, 1: 11-16.
65. Portugal, D., Smith, J. *Myocarditis and the athlete.* In: Sudden Cardiac Death in the Athlete. Estes, N.A.M., Salem, D.N., Wang, P.J. Futura Media Service: Armonk 1998: 349-71.
66. Angelini, A., Basso, C., Turrini, P., Thiene, G. *Clinical and pathological relevance of endomyocardial biopsy.* In: Arrhythmogenic Right Ventricular Cardiomyopathy/Dysplasia. Nava A., Rossi L., Thiene G. (Eds.). Elsevier Science B.V.: Amsterdam 1997, 257-68.
67. Furlanello, F., Bettini, R., Cozzi F. et al. *Ventricular arrhythmias and sudden death in athletes. Clinical aspects of life-threatening arrhythmias.* Ann NY Acad Sci 1984, 427: 253-79.
68. Furlanello, F., Bettini, R., Vergara, G. et al. *Markers and trigger mechanismo of sudden cardiac death.* In: Sudden Cardiac Death. Bayes de Luna, A., Brugada, P., Cosin Aguilar, J., Navarro-Lopez, F. (Eds.). Kluwer Academic Publishers: Dordrecht 1990, 87-98.
69. Furlanello, F., Bertoldi, A., Galassi, A. et al. *Management of severe cardiac arrhythmic events in elite athletes.* PACE 1999, 22 (Part II), A 165.

CHAPTER 8

ARRHYTHMIAS IN SPECIAL SITUATIONS

P. Ferrés[1], F. Drago[2], A. Biffi[3], R. Elosua[4], M.T. Subirana[1],
A. Aguilar[1], F. Sardella[3], A. Dal Monte[3] and A. Bayés de Luna[1]
*[1]Department of Cardiology and Cardiac Surgery, Hospital de la Santa
Creu i Sant Pau, Barcelona, Spain, [2]Department of Pediatric Cardiac
Sugery, Ospedale Pediatrico Bambino Gesú, Rome, Italy, [3]Sports Science
Institute, Italian National Olympic Committee, Rome, Italy and [4]Lipids
and Cardiovascular Epidemiology Unit, Institut Municipal d'Investigació
Médica, Barcelona, Spain.*

In this chapter we will review and briefly discuss some aspects related to arrhythmias and
exposure to certain special situations (high altitudes or underwater activities) as well as
in special athletic populations (veterans or pediatrics).

Arrhythmia at High Altitudes (Mountain Climbing)

Cardiovascular and respiratory adaptations to exposure of the human organism to altitudes greater than 3,500-4,000 meters have been the subject of numerous scientific studies. These have been carried out on the mountain itself, as well as in the laboratory, by
simulating heights similar to those of the Himalayan peaks (1, 2).

The reduction in partial pressure of oxygen in the inhaled air is the primary factor conditioning the reduction of functional capacity at high altitudes (3). This low partial pressure of oxygen produces a reduction in the saturation of oxygen of the hemoglobin and,
consequently, hypoxemia. The organism increases the plasmatic concentration of the
hemoglobin and the capacity to liberate oxygen by increasing 2,3-diphosphoglycerate.

In serious exposure to hypoxia, the heart works 15% faster at submaximum workload
as a consequence of the increase in the plasma concentration of catecholamines and its
effect on heart rate (4). On the other hand, maximum heart rate decreases at heights of
3,000-3,500 meters and at heights greater than 5,000 meters it seems to not be able to
register more than 155-160 beats/min (5) (Fig. 1). According to Cerretelli (6), if exposure
is prolonged over several weeks, maximal wear on the heart under stress is reduced up to
15% at 5,000 meters and up to 30% at 5,800 meters, due to reduction of the cardiac pre-
load, increase in the arterial-pulmonary pressure and severe hypoxia (7).

Despite the fat that with hypoxia plasma catecholamines are increased, adrenergic
receptors are desensitized and the sensitivity of muscarinic receptors (parasympathetic) is

A. Bayés de Luna et al. (eds.), Arrhythmias and Sudden Death in Athletes, 107–118.

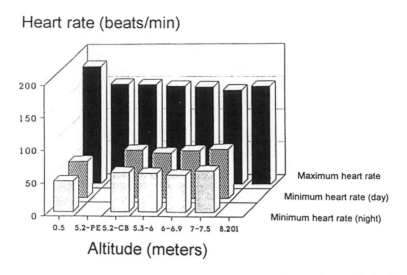

Heart rate (beats/min)

Altitude (meters)

Maximum heart rate

Minimum heart rate (day)

Minimum heart rate (night)

Figure 1. Maximum, minimum day-time and night-time heart rate behavior at different altitudes. Reproduced with permission from (72).

increased, the result is a lower maximal heart rate under stress (and pharmacology) than that recorded at sea level (8). These effects are partially reversible by administering atropine (9). However, the heart rate at rest and during sleep tends to be slightly higher than that recorded at sea level (10), although severe bradyarrhythmia can also be observed at rest and mainly during sleep. Using Holter monitoring, some investigators have registered pauses of up to 7-8 seconds per second and third degree atrioventricular block (10, 11) (Fig. 2).

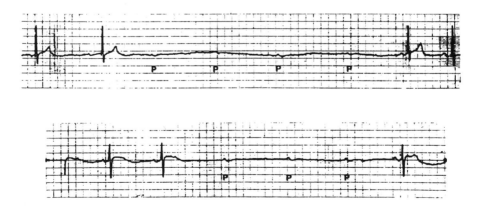

Figure 2. Eight-second cardiac arrest due to complete atrioventricular block in a mountain climber at 8,201 meters. Reproduced with permission from (72).

Other commonly described arrhythmias include increases in ventricular and supraventricular automatism, with isolated premature compounds being more frequent. More prolonged periods of bigeminy, especially related to age (12), have also been described.

The increase in ventricular automatism seems to be reduced by adaptation to intermittent high altitude hypoxia (13).

Arterial-pulmonary hypertension developed at high altitudes is one of the factors conditioning cardiovascular adaptations to high altitudes. This increase in pulmonary pressure seems to be due to several factors: the low temperature and barometric pressure unleash vasoconstriction, which hypoxia increases. At the same time, vascular permeability increases and the plaque's ability to aggregate and coagulate is altered. This causes an increase in vascular-pulmonary resistance (14, 15), which is the physiopathologic base for pulmonary edema at great heights, especially in individuals who are predisposed due to a constitutional factor that makes them prone to develop pulmonary edema (16). Electric alterations that convert into an increase in pressure in right cavities, increasing the extent of P-waves in V1-V2 and negative T-waves in right precordia have also been described. These changes are very marked in cases of pulmonary edema (17, 18).

Arrhythmia when Practicing Underwater Sports

There are two main types of underwater sport: scuba diving and sports practiced through apnea immersion or by holding one's breath. This latter group could also include synchronized swimming. In the United States, it has been calculated that more than five million people practice some type of underwater sport (19). In this chapter we examine the heart rate response and the prevalence of arrhythmias during underwater sports in humans. Furthermore, we illustrate our personal experience in this field. The reduction in heart rate (bradycardia) that has been observed in response to apneic immersion is considered to be a component of an oxygen-conserving mechanism termed the mammalian dive reflex (20). This reflex is accompanied by some cardiac modifications, such as vagal bradycardia, due to depression of sympathetic activity and peripheral vasoconstriction. It is argued that the only well-demonstrated response to apnea that humans share with other diving species is bradycardia (21). Investigations of apneic heart rate in humans and explanations for the responses observed are many and varied. A bradycardic response to apnea at rest is reasonably well established, with a more pronounced reduction in heart rate occurring during apneic facial or whole body immersion than during breath-holding on land. Some studies found that bradycardia on immersion persisted in humans in spite of vigorous underwater swimming (22). These data could be explained by an interaction between the vagal and the sympathetic nervous systems, whereby adrenergic tone may be directly reduced by an increase in vagal tone (23). Much of the literature would contend that the onset of bradycardia is immediate upon apnea, prompting the conclusion that the changes in heart rate are so rapid they could only be initiated by reflexes (24). Prolongation of the diastolic phase, together with the disappearance or fluttering of P-waves accompanies the slowing of the heart rate during apneic bradycardia.

Apneic heart rate is determined by a number of variables and the alteration of one or a combination of these may produce quite different results. Factors implicated in the phenomenon of apneic bradycardia include the influence of the temperature and physical conditions of the individual, varying lung volumes, depth of immersion in water, body position during the apneic episode and the psychological state of the individual (25). A number of researchers showed that apneic bradycardia are temperature-dependent. In fact, cold temperatures, particularly with regard to facial immersion, are said to potentiate a reduction in heart rate (26). The most efficient range in producing bradycardia was described as being between 15-25 °C. The rest of the body, in contrast, requires a longer period of time to make the same adaptations. Concerning physical conditions and underwater experience, there is a general agreement that the greatest bradycardiac response is seen in competent underwater divers (27). The apparent relationship between experience in underwater apneic activity and the extent of bradycardia has been ascribed to a greater breath holding capacity due to changes in lung volumes and a tolerance to increased carbon dioxide tensions brought about by regular underwater training (27). Few studies have investigated the specific effects of age upon heart rate during breath holding. The majority of those that have, however, support the view that young age potentiates apnea-induced bradycardia. Gooden (28) postulated that in the human fetus, such cardiovascular adjustments constitute a protective mechanism against asphyxia during birth and that for this reason young infants may retain a particularly sensitive "diving reflex". Furthermore, the influence of varying lung volumes has been implicated in the findings of several authors, with the majority contending that large lung volumes potentiate apneic bradycardia (29). Lower heart rates were noted in subjects with larger lung volumes, prompting the conclusion that relative vital capacity was a determinant of the magnitude of bradycardia during apnea. Bonneau *et al.* (30, 31) used Holter electrocardiogram (ECG) monitoring to study the electrocardiographic findings in a group of divers. For 70% of the cases, bradycardia was associated with isolated supraventricular ectopic beats or, more frequently, with multiple salvas. Ventricular ectopic beats were also frequently recorded and were usually bigeminal. Ishikawa *et al.* (32) also found a high percentage of arrhythmias in a group of 64 children who were monitored while diving: 44 of them (69%) showed some form of bradyarrhythmia or tachyarrhythmia during immersion.

PERSONAL EXPERIENCE

In our Institute of Sports Science of the Italian National Olympic Committee, both with regard to routine evaluation tests for national team athletes as well as research protocols, we used especially designed specific ergometers (33). One of the latest ergometers, designed by Dal Monte, is an ergometric pool. Such a sophisticated piece of equipment has greatly fostered the ergometry of some sports that until recently involved environmental-objective evaluation problems such as swimming, canoeing, wind surfing and underwater sports. Our aim was to establish the involvement of the heart and the metabolic demand of some trained subjects during maximal apnea in the ergometric pool and to compare the results with those of a test carried out with scuba diving. The ergometric pool consists of an open-air water conduit measuring 7 x 3 meters where the water, lined up by four special grilles, is set into motion by means of four propellers thrust by a 240

HP marine engine. The flowing speed of the water reaches 7 m/sec at maximum. The pool is fitted with a special side glass enabling the researchers to evaluate the underwater behavior of the athletes and material involved. In studies on apnea performed in the ergometric pool, we wish to emphasize that the tests were carried out under low-risk conditions for the subjects being tested, as the center was fully equipped to deal with any medical emergency, should the need have arisen.

Twenty-five athletes (20 males and five females) practicing apnea diving at a competitive level, mean age 27 ± 4.3 years, were tested. During the medical examination, which was required to evaluate the subjects' eligibility for sports activity, none of the athletes showed any general pathologic conditions or electrocardiographic alteration or arrhythmia. The test included: i) "dry" apnea: the athlete, lying supine was requested to perform maximal apnea and continuous ECG was recorded throughout the test; ii) Valsalva maneuver; iii) apnea test in water: athletes performed the maximal apnea, after a 30 sec voluntary hyperventilation, finning at a speed of 0.754 meters/sec in water at a temperature of 26 °C; iii) measurement of lactic acid level in the blood; and iv) test with scuba: this test was carried out the day after the previous test. Similarly, surface electrodes were used for monitoring heart activity. The athletes, on wearing a scuba diving apparatus, were made to start a test whereby they had to swim with flippers for 12 min at the same speed used for the apnea test.

The results showed a strong bradycardia, often lower than 40 beats/min, in all athletes during the apnea test. One athlete, in the final stage of apnea, reached a heart rate of 28 beats/min. Furthermore, in relation to maximum bradycardia, 86.7% of athletes had some type of cardiac tachyarrhythmias during water apnea. In contrast, only 13% of the subjects showed cardiac arrhythmias during "dry" apnea and 7% during the scuba diving test. Various degrees of ventricular as well as supraventricular arrhythmias were recorded. Two athletes showed ventricular couplets and triplets at the end of apnea (Table 1). It is difficult to explain the pathogenic mechanism underlying this high prevalence of cardiac arrhythmias during underwater diving. Probably, sinus bradycardia may *per se* increase the dispersion of the ventricular refractoriness and, therefore, increase the possibility of the reentry phenomenon (34). Furthermore, increased vagal tone mediated by muscarinic receptors shortens atrial refractory periods and can facilitate the occurrence of atrial tachyarrhythmias (35). This study is in agreement with other studies that showed a greater occurrence of arrhythmias in underwater conditions than in out of water ones. This suggests that arrhythmias could be one of the possible causes of accidents during diving. Probably, the increase of hydrostatic pressure causes an increase in the blood volume and an expansion of the heart's chambers, in particular, that of the right ventricle, which could serve as an arrhythmogenic mechanism during underwater sports (36).

Table 1. Prevalence of cardiac arrhythmias during apnea.

	Heart rate (beats/min)		Arrhythmias (%)	Length (sec)
	Start	End		
"Dry" apnea	114 ± 22	68 ± 8	13.3	183 ± 62
Underwater apnea	119 ± 22	50 ± 13	86.7	85 ± 20
Statistics	NS	$p < 0.005$	$p < 0.001$	—

RECOMMENDATIONS

Since the greater occurrence of arrhythmias is at the final stage of apnea diving, the limit of apnea should not be prolonged. Cardiac arrhythmias could facilitate underwater syncope, which is generally induced by "hypoxy neuron syndrome". Therefore, an in-depth cardiovascular examination should be mandatory in athletes engaged in underwater sports. In particular, subjects with complex forms of arrhythmias on land should be excluded from apnea diving. Twenty-four-hour Holter ECG monitoring including a training session could be very useful. Furthermore, divers with previous experience of syncope during underwater apnea should undergo a tilting-test to reproduce symptoms. Echocardiogram (and possibly transesophageal pacing as well) may be very useful in identifying patent foramen ovale, one of the important causes of neurological symptoms during decompression illness in scuba divers (arterial gas embolism from the right to the left side of the heart).

Arrhythmias in Senior Athletes

Current trends in fitness and the proven benefits of regular physical activity on the cardiovascular system and on the organism in general has made it more and more common to have an increasing amount of men and women over the age of 65-70 years taking part in sports. Specifically, we will refer to the most extreme examples of this phenomenon: very senior long-distance and marathon runners who actively participate in popular races, cross-country races and even marathons that require them to be remarkably well-trained, with many of them doing weekly runs of over 50 km.

Despite the exceedingly small risk of sudden cardiac death associated with marathon running (37), it is well known that coronary artery disease is the most frequent cause of sudden death in athletes older than 35 years (38-42).

With physiological aging, the prevalence and complexity of hyperkinetic arrhythmia (43, 44) increases significantly and bradyarrhythmia is also more frequently found (45). Fleg and Kennedy (46) studied the prevalence of arrhythmia in 98 healthy men and women aged 60-85 years and found a low rate of bradyarrhythmias (ventricular rates less than 40 times/min or asystolia for longer than 1.5 sec). Regarding hyperkinetic arrhythmia, they observed that the prevalence of frequent ventricular and supraventricular ectopic beats (>100/24 h) was 17% and 26%, respectively; they documented ventricular couplets in 11% and ventricular tachycardia in 4%. Bjerregaard (47) found a similar prevalence of ventricular arrhythmia in a healthy population of 76 men and women aged 60-70 years.

Senior athletes have a greater prevalence of complex ventricular arrhythmia. They also present more significant bradycardia during nighttime rest than healthy sedentary people of their age. Jensen-Urstad *et al.* (48) used 48-h Holter monitoring in 11 senior male athletes aged 68-77 years (average age 73) and compared them with a control group of 12 sedentary or moderately active individuals. The prevalence of ventricular arrhythmia was significantly higher in the athletes, given that nine of the 11 athletes presented polymorphic premature ventricular complexes, couplets or ventricular tachycardia (one case), while in only five of the 12 control individuals was this arhythmia recorded. Regarding bradyarrhythmia (Fig. 3), seven of the 11 athletes showed ventricular rates below 40 times/min at some point during the night, which did not occur in any of the control group. Two athletes presented asystolia for more than 2 sec: in one case 2.3 sec due to sinoauricular blocking and in the other 2.6 sec due to second-degree atrioventricular block. Also, two athletes and one control individual presented intermittent second degree atrioventricular block during nighttime rest. The authors conclude that the higher prevalence of ventricular arrhythmia and bradycardia in the group of senior athletes than in the control group could increase the risk of sudden death (48), although no follow-up was made.

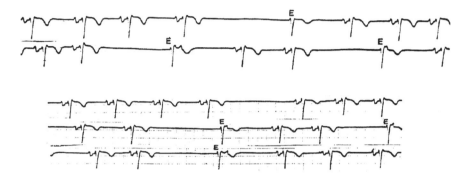

Figure 3. Holter monitoring in a 60-year-old runner: sinus bradycardia and atrioventricular junction beats (E) at rest.

On the other hand, positive modifications in R-R variability can partially offset the risk of malignant ventricular arrhythmia. R-R variability decreases with age (49), making older patients more susceptible to malignant ventricular arrhythmia. In the same study (48), the group of senior athletes presented greater R-R variability than did the control group, which suggests that intense physical activity can delay the age at which reduced R-R variability is recorded and can also reduce the risk of presenting a malignant ventricular arrhythmia.

The existence of sinusal pauses of up to 12 sec in an asymptomatic senior athlete has also been documented (50), which gives rise to the need for pacemakers in extreme cases, given the possibility of developing neurological lesions, malignant ventricular arrhythmia and sudden death.

Arrhythmia in the Pediatric Athlete Population

Playing sports has become globalized over recent years and this is especially true of children; in fact, the large number of children and adolescents under the age of 16 years who regularly participate in sports training and competitions constitutes a social phenomenon. Also, early specialization and the significant reduction in the age of maximum performance in numerous sports (gymnastics, swimming, tennis) have produced a remarkable load in training and competition for children and adolescents. They are still growing and these intense physical demands could favor the appearance of dysrhythmia and sudden death in this subgroup.

Unexpected sudden death in apparently healthy children is very infrequent, occuring in about 1.3-8.5 children for every 100,000 patients/year (51). It generally occurs in children with undiagnosed heart murmur, which only appears in the case of sudden death. Driscoll (52) studied 63 cases of unexpected sudden death in children and found that 35 (55%) presented hypertrophic cardiomyopathy, 15 (24%) had congenital coronary abnormalities, six (10%) showed aortic stenosis and in only two cases (3%) was no cause found. Prior syncope is the main clinical manifestation of possible underlying cardiopathy. In the group studied by Driscoll, this was present in up to a third of the cases. Importantly, death came about at the time physical effort was being exerted in two-thirds of the cases. This shows the importance of detecting heart disease in asymptomatic, apparently healthy children who regularly play a sport and of properly evaluating any child who shows syncopal symptoms when practicing a sport. Other researchers, such as Denfield and Garson (53), have also found other etiologies responsible for sudden death during physical effort: myocarditis (9%), long Q-T syndrome, Wolff-Parkinson-White syndrome and aortic rupture with Marfan's syndrome. Niimura and Maki (54) studied 62 children who had suddenly died during physical activity. Of these, 18 children had cardiovascular disease and in nine, postmortem examination showed hypertrophic cardiomyopathy in three cases, myocarditis in three, Kawasaki disease in two and long Q-T syndrome in one.

Regarding the young population with cardiac disease, it is not true that most patients died suddenly during exercise. In fact, Lambert (55) reported that sudden death was related to exercise in about 10% and Garson (56) found sudden cardiac death in 22% of the patient population studied.

Another pediatric subgroup to keep in mind are children with congenital cardiopathies who have had successful operations and live normal lives, including playing sports in many instances, despite the fact that in most cases we recommend avoiding competitive sports. The possibility of ventricular tachyarrhythmia is especially relevant in children who have undergone Fallot tetralogy or large vessel transposition (57).

Complete atrioventricular block, whether congenital or acquired (surgery, ablation) is another entity which presents problems to sports players (58). When the right maximal rate of escape rhythm with effort is achieved, and no ventricular ectopies are documented, physicians can be more permissive about authorizing the practice of sports. If this does not occur, sports should be restricted, especially at a competitive level and every case requires periodic evaluation for the implantation of a permanent pacemaker (Fig. 4). Also, severe ventricular ectopy may appear with an increased risk of sudden death, especially in individuals with coexisting Q-T prolongation (59).

Supraventricular arrhythmias are rarely a cause of sudden death in the pediatric athletic population. The majority of supraventricular paroxysmal tachycardia is caused be a reentry mechanism due to there being an accessory pathway. At present it tends to be definitively treated in children and adolescents by means of ablation with radiofrequency (60). In Wolf-Parkinson-White syndrome, this eliminates the accessory pathway that

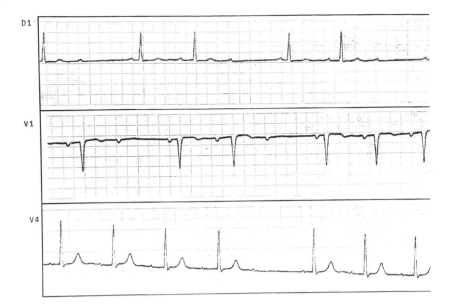

Figure 4. High-level 13-year-old swimmer: second degree atrioventricular block type Mobitz I.

permits tachycardia with very high ventricular frequencies and in the case of auricular fibrillation, especially during exercise, the risk of ventricular fibrillation and sudden death (61, 62). Crises of vagal-originated paroxysmic auricular fibrillation in children are rare. However, if detected, the proper steps should be taken to prevent them (63). Atrial tachycardia and atrial flutter are frequent late postoperative sequelae and may be responsible for sudden death during physical activity in children with complex congenital heart disease who have required extensive atrial surgery, such as Mustard, Senning or Fontan procedures (64, 65).

Ventricular tachyarrhythmias can degenerate, especially during physical exercise, into ventricular fibrillation and sudden death. This is especially important in patients with hypertrophic cardiomyopathy, the most frequent cause of sudden death in children and young adults (42). Malignant ventricular arrhythmias are also the first cause of sudden death in the other heart diseases in children: arrhythmogenic substrate in myocarditis (66), long Q-T syndrome (67) or arrhythmogenic right ventricular dysplasia (68). Finally, myocardial ischemia may be the mechanism responsible for malignant arrhythmias in congenital coronary abnormalities (69), Kawasaki disease (70) and severe aortic stenosis (71).

References

1. Sleep, M.K., Rock, P.B., Young, P.M., Houston, C.S. *Operation Everest II: Elevated high-altitude pulmonary resistance unresponsive to oxygen.* J Appl Physiol 1987, 63(2): 521-30.
2. Reeves, J.T., Groves, B.M., Sutton, J.R., et al. *Operation Everest II: Preservation of cardiac function at extreme altitude.* J Appl Physiol 1987, 63(2): 531-9.

3.   Cerretelli, P. *Gas exchange at high altitude.* In: Pulmonary Gas Exchange. Academic Press: New York 1980, 97-147.
4.   Sutton, J.R., Jones, N.L. *Exercise at altitude.* Ann Rev Physiol 1983, 45: 427-37.
5.   Karlinae, J.S., Sarnquist, F.F., Graber, D.J., Peters, R.M., West, J.B. *The electrocardiogram at extreme altitude: Experience on Mt Everest.* Am Heart J 1985, 109: 505-13.
6.   Cerretelli, P., Di Prampero, P.E. *Aerobic and anaerobic metabolism during exercise at altitude.* Med Sport Sci 1985, 19: 1-19.
7.   Suarez, J., Alexander, J.K., Houston, C.S. *Enhanced left ventricular systolic performance at high altitude during operation Everest II.* Am J Cardiol 1987, 60: 137-42.
8.   Richalet, J.P., Kacimi, R., Antezana, A.M. *The control of cardiac chronotropic function in hypobaric hypoxia.* Int J Sports Med 1992, 13(1): 22-4.
9.   Hartley, L., Vogel, J., Cruz, J. *Reduction of maximal exercise heart rate at altitude and its reversal with atropine.* J Appl Physiol 1974, 36: 326-65.
10.   Serra, J.R., Martínez Ferrer, R., Elosua, R., Garido, E. *Adaptación cardiovascular en situaciones especiales.* In: Cardiología Deportiva. A. Bayés de Luna, et al. (Eds.). Mosby/Doyma Libros: Barcelona 1994, 106-18.
11.   Weil, J.V., Kryger, M.H., Scoggin, C.H. *Sleep and breathing at high altitude.* In: C. Guilleminault, W.C. Demnt (Eds.). Sleep Apnea Syndromes. Alan R Liss Inc.: New York 1978.
12.   Alexander, J.K. *Age, altitude and arrhythmias.* Tex Heart Inst J 1995, 22(4): 308-16.
13.   Meerson, F.Z., Ustinova, E.E., Orlova, E.H. *Prevention and elimination of heart arrhythmias by adaptation to intermittent high altitude hypoxia.* Clin Cardiol 1987, 10: 783-9.
14.   Gray, G.W. *High altitude pulmonary edema.* Sem Resp Med 1983, 5: 141-50.
15.   West, J.B., Mathieu-Costello, O. *High altitude pulmonary edema is caused by stress failure of pulmonary capillaries.* Int J Sports Med 1992, 13 (1): 54-8.
16.   Yagi, H., Yamada, H., Kobayashi, T., Sekiguchi, M. *Doppler assessment of pulmonary hypertension induced by hypoxic breathing in subjects susceptible to high altitude pulmonary edema.* Am Rev Respir Dis 1990, 142: 796-801.
17.   Karlinae, J.S., Sarnquist, F.F., Garber, D.J., Peters, R.N., West, J.B. *The electrocardiogram at extreme altitude: Experience on Mt Everest.* Am Heart J 1985, 109: 505-13.
18.   Fiorenzano, G., Papalia, M.A., Parravicini, M., Rastelli, V., Bigi, R., Dottorini, M. *Prolonged ECG abnormalities in a subject with high altitude pulmonary edema.* J Sports Med Phys Fitness, 1997, 37(4): 292-6.
19.   Melamed, Y., Shupak, A., Bitterman, H. *Medical problems associated with underwater diving.* N Engl J Med 1992, 326: 30-5.
20.   Asmussen, E., Kristiansson, N.G. *The "diving bradycardia" in exercising man.* Acta Physiologica Scandinavica 1965, 73: 527-35.
21.   Craig, A.B. *Heart rate responses to apneic underwater diving and to breath-holding in man.* J Appl Physiol 1963, 18: 854-62.
22.   Irving, L. *Bradycardia in human divers.* J Appl Physiol 1963, 18: 489-91.
23.   Finley, J.P., Bonet, J.F., Waxman, M.B. *Autonomic pathways responsible for bradycardia on facial immersion.* J Appl Physiol 1979, 47: 1218-22.
24.   Bove, A.A., Lynch, P.R., Connel, J.V., Harding, J.M. *Diving reflex after physical training.* J Appl Physiol 1968, 25: 70-2.
25.   Manley, L. *Apneic heart rate response in humans. A review.* Sports Medicine 1990, 9: 286-310.
26.   Hong, S.K. *Thermal considerations.* In: Schilling (Ed.). The Physician's Guide to Diving Medicine. Plenum Press: New York 1984.
27.   Oldridge, N.B., Heigenhauser, G.J.F., Sutton, J.R., Jones, N.L. *Resting and exercise heart rate with apnoea and facial immersion in female swimmers.* J Appl Physiol 1978, 45: 875-83.
28.   Gooden, B.A. *Drowning and the diving reflex in man.* Med J Austral 1972, 2: 583-7.
29.   Magel, J.R., McArdle, W.D., Weiss, N.L., Stone, S., Newman, A. *Heart rate response to apnea and face immersion.* J Sports Med Phys Fitness 1982, 22: 135-46.
30.   Bonneau, A., Friemel, F. *Arrhythmia and vago-sympathetic equilibrium in athletic divers.* Arch Mal Coeur Vaiss 1989, 82: 99-105.
31.   Bonneau, A., Friemel, F., Lapierre, D. *Electrocardiographic aspects of skin diving.* Eur J Appl Physiol 1989, 58: 487-93.

32. Ishikawa, H., Matsushima, M., Nagashima, M., Osuga, A. *Screening of children with arrhythmias for arrhythmia development during diving and swimming-face immersion as a substitute for diving and exercise stress testing as a substitute for swimming.* Jpn Circ J 1992, 56: 881-90.

33. Dal Monte, A., Faccini, P., Biffi, A., Faina, M. *Specific ergometry in the maximum stimulation of cardiac activity.* New Trend Arrhyth 1988, 7: 163-9.

34. Brachman, J. *Bradycardia dependent triggered activity: Relevance to drug-induced multiform ventricular tachycardia.* Circulation 1983, 65: 546-50.

35. Prystowsky, E.N. *Enhanced vagal tone shortens atrial refractoriness in man.* Am J Cardiol 1983, 51: 96-100.

36. Mc Donough, J.R., Barytt, J.P., Saffron, J.C. Letter to Editor. N Engl J Med 1992, 326(22): 1498.

37. Maron, B.J., Poliac, L.C., Roberts, W.O. *Risk for sudden cardiac death associated with marathon running.* J Am Coll Cardiol 1996, 28(2): 428-31.

38. Kenny, A., Shapiro, L.M. *Sudden cardiac death in athletes.* Br Med Bull 1992, 48 (3): 534-45.

39. Thompson, P.D. *Athletes, athletics, and sudden cardiac death.* Med Sci Sports Exerc 1993, 25(9): 981-4.

40. Wight, J.N. Jr., Salem, D. *Sudden cardiac death and the athlete's heart.* Arch Intern Med 1995, 155(14): 1473-80.

41. Jensen-Urstad, M. *Sudden death and physical activity in athletes and nonathletes.* Scand J Med Sci Sports 1995, 5(5): 279-84.

42. Maron, B.J., Shirani, J., Poliac, L.C., Mathenge, R., Roberts, W.C., Mueller, F.O. *Sudden death in young competitive athletes. Clinical, demographic, and pathological profiles.* JAMA 1996, 276: 199-204.

43. Kantelip, J.P., Sage, E., Duchene-Marullaz, P. *Findings on ambulatory electrocardiographic monitoring in subjects older than 80 years.* Am J Cardiol 1986, 57: 398.

44. Marcus, F.I., Ruskin, J.N., Surawitz, B. *Arrhythmias.* J Am Coll Cardiol 1987, 10(2): 66.

45. Pfeiffer, M.A., Weinberg, C.R., Cook, D. *Differential changes of autonomic nervous system function with age in man.* Am J Med 1983, 75: 249.

46. Fleg, J.L., Kennedy, H.L. *Cardiac arrhythmias in a healthy elderly population: Detection by 24 hour ambulatory electrocardiography.* Chest 1982, 81: 302-7.

47. Bjerregaard, P. *Premature beats in healthy subjects 40-79 years of age.* Eur Heart J 1982, 3: 493-503.

48. Jensen-Urstad, K., Bouvier, F., Saltin, B., Jensen-Urstad, M. *High prevalence of arrhythmias in elderly male athletes with a lifelong history of regular strenuous exercise.* Heart 1998, 79: 161-4.

49. Bigger, T.J. Jr., Fleiss, J.L., Steinman, R.C., et al. *RR variability in healthy, middle-aged persons compared with patients with chronic coronary heart disease or recent acute myocardial infarction.* Circulation 1995, 91: 1936-43.

50. Northcote, R.J., Rankin, A.C., Scullion, R., Logan, W. *Is severe bradycardia in veteran athletes an indication for a permanent pacemaker?* Br Med J 1989, 298: 231.

51. Silka, M.J., Kron, J., Wallance, G.C., Cutler, J.E., McAnulty, J.H. *Assessment and follw-up of pediatric survivors of sudden cardiac death.* Circulation 1990, 82: 341-9.

52. Driscoll, D.J. *Sudden, unexpected death in children and adolescents.* J Am Coll Cardiol 1985, 5 (Suppl.): 118-21.

53. Denfield, S.W., Garson, A. Jr. *Sudden death in children and young adults.* Pediatr Clin North Am 1990, 37: 215-31.

54. Niimura, I., Maki, T. *Sudden cardiac death in childhood.* Jpn Circ J 1989, 53: 1571-80.

55. Lambert, E.C., Menon, V.A., Wagner, H.R., Vlad, P. *Sudden unexpected death from cardiovascular disease in children.* Am J Cardiol 1974, 34: 89-96.

56. Garson, A. Jr. *Sudden death in a pediatric cardiology population, 1958 to 1983: Relation to prior arrhythmias.* J Am Coll Cardiol 1985, 5 (Suppl.): 138-41.

57. Gillette, P.C., Garson, A. Jr. *Sudden cardiac death in the pediatric population.* Circulation 1992, 85 (Suppl. I): 64–9.

58. Serra Grima, J.R., Subirana, M.T., Bayés de Luna, A.J. *Recomendaciones para la práctica deportiva en pacientes con cardiopatía.* In: A. Bayés de Luna, et al. (Eds.). Cardiología Deportiva. Mosby/Doyma Libros: Barcelona, 1994, 155-171.

59. Winkler, R.B., Freed, M.D., Nadas, A.S. *Exercise-induced ventricular ectopy in children and young adults with complete heart block.* Am Heart J 1980, 99: 87-92.

60. Maron, B.J., Mitchell, J.H. *26ᵗʰ Bethesda Conference: Recommendations for determining eligibility for competition in athletes with cardiovascular abnormalities.* J Am Coll Cardiol 1994, 24(4): 845-99.
61. Furlanello, F., Ferrés, P., Bertoldi, A., et al. *Muerte súbita en el deportista.* In: Cardiología Deportiva. A.Bayés de Luna, et al. (Eds.). Mosby/Doyma Libros: Barcelona 1994, 84-93.
62. Deal, B.J., Dick, M., Beerman, L. *Cardiac arrest in young patients with Wolff-Parkinson-White Syndrome.* Pacing Clin Electrophysiol 1995, 18: 815.
63. Bayés de Luna, A.J. Clinical Electrocardiography: A Textbook. Futura Publishing Co.: New York 1993.
64. Haines, D.R., Di Marco, J.P. *Sustained intraatrial reentrant tachycardia: Clinical, electrocardiographic and electrophysiologic characteristics and long term follow up.* J Am Coll Cardiol 1990, 15: 1345-54.
65. Garson, A., Bink-Boelkens, M., Hesslein, P.S., Hordof, A.J., Keane, J.F., Neches, W.H. *Atrial flutter in the young: A collaborative study of 380 cases.* J Am Coll Cardiol 1993, 71: 122-4.
66. Friedman, R.A., Kearney, D.L., Moak, J.P., Fenrich, A.L., Parry, J.C. *Persistence of ventricular arrhythmia after resolution of occult myocarditis in children and young adults.* J Am Coll Cardiol 1994, 24: 780-3.
67. Garson, A. Jr., Dick, M., Fournier, A., et al. *The long QT syndrome in children. An international study of 287 patients.* Circulation 1993, 87(6): 1866-72.
68. Daliento, R., Turrini, P., Nava, A., et al. *Arrhythmogenic right ventricular cardiomyopathy in young versus adults patients: Similarities and differences.* J Am Coll Cardiol 1995, 25: 655-64.
69. Lipsett, J., Byard, R.W., Carpenter, B.F., Jimenez, C.L., Bourne, A.J. *Anomalous coronary arteries arising from the aorta associated with sudden death in infancy and early childhood: An autopsy series.* Arch Pathol Lab Med 1991, 115(8): 770-3.
70. Burns, J.C., Shike, H., Gordon, J.B., Kawasaki, T. *Sequelae of Kawasaki disease in adolescents and young adults.* J Am Coll Cardiol 1996, 28(1): 253-7.
71. Perchet, H., Gaudeau, S., Casasoprana, A., Corone, P., Castaigne, A., Vernant, P. *Valvotomy and congenital aortic valve stenosis: Long-term results.* Arch Mal Coeur Vaiss 1991, 84(5): 705-10.
72. Martínez Ferrer, J. Adaptación Humana a la Extrema Altura. Instituto Municipal del Deporte Vitoria-Gasteiz (Spain) 1990.

CHAPTER 9

GUIDELINES FOR COMPETITIVE ATHLETES WITH ARRHYTHMIAS

T. Al-Sheikh and D.P. Zipes
*Krannert Institute of Cardiology, Indiana University School of Medicine
and the Roudebush Veterans Administration Medical Center,
Indianapolis, Indiana, USA*

General Considerations

Guidelines for athletic participation are needed to recognize athletes at risk for arrhythmias and to prevent sudden cardiac death and reduce the risk for arrhythmia-related morbidity. Few available data exist that have been obtained from well-designed, prospective studies to determine whether certain arrhythmias increase the athlete's risk for sudden death or cause significant symptoms, such as syncope or presyncope. It is often difficult to determine the significance of a specific cardiac rhythm disturbance in assessing an athlete's eligibility for competitive sports. Sudden cardiac death is rare in young people (1, 2); its incidence is estimated to be <1% of that in adults (3). Nonetheless, a significant proportion of these deaths occurs in relation to exercise. Death related to sports is always a shocking event and the recent premature and sudden cardiac deaths of elite athletes have focused attention on athletes with known arrhythmias (4).

Heavy physical training produces different functional and morphological cardiac changes. Athletes differ from untrained individuals in many respects and are considered a distinct group. Practically all types of arrhythmias have been observed in athletes and it is not unusual to discover an arrhythmia during routine evaluation, which can sometimes create a dilemma regarding proper workup and management. Arrhythmias are often unpredictable and may not occur in the athlete during each sporting event. Factors related to the autonomic nervous system probably play a major role in determining whether an arrhythmia occurs, as well as the rate and effect of the arrhythmia on hemodynamic responses and symptoms (5). Symptoms and their effects may vary depending on the type of sporting activity. The same arrhythmia may minimally affect a competitive golfer but severely incapacitate any other athlete, such as cross-country skiers performing at peak physical effort.

It is important to understand the range of normal heart rate and rhythm for the trained athlete (6, 7): heart rate of 25 beats/min and sinus pauses lasting >2 seconds may be found on 24-h Holter ambulatory electrocardiographic (ECG) recordings. Type I second-degree atrioventricular (AV) block and single uniform premature ventricular complexes, couplets and nonsustained ventricular tachycardia are uncommon (7).

A. Bayés de Luna et al. (eds.), Arrhythmias and Sudden Death in Athletes, 119–151.

Recommendations and guidance need to be balanced between an effort to avoid unduly restricting activity and the hope of reducing the risk of death and injury due to a rhythm disturbance.

Despite the lack of certain information, some firm conclusions can be reached. Certain arrhythmias create symptoms and are dangerous in and of themselves regardless of the clinical situation in which they occur (8). These arrhythmias are generally characterized by very rapid or very slow heart rates that significantly compromise cardiac output and coronary or cerebral blood flow. Certain persistent tachyarrhythmias can affect cardiac function and cause a cardiomyopathy (9). Bradyarrhythmias in athletes are most often found at rest and usually do not produce any clinical symptoms. These arrhythmias are generally benign and they almost always reflect enhanced vagal tone.

Athletes with coronary heart disease (10), hypertrophic cardiomyopathy (11, 12), arrhythmogenic right ventricular dysplasia (13), aortic stenosis (14) and other forms of congenital heart disease (1) are probably at greater risk for cardiac arrest and sudden death during and just after exercise. This is probably true whether or not arrhythmias have been recognized previously (15-17). In general, athletes with symptoms possibly related to cardiac arrhythmias, such as syncope, near syncope and palpitations, should be carefully evaluated before being permitted to participate in competitive sports. A consideration of cardiac hemodynamic status is critical because right or left ventricular dysfunction is an additional important predictor of arrhythmic death (18, 19). The presence of a significant rhythm disturbance in athletes with abnormal cardiac hemodynamic status (from any cause unrelated to the arrhythmia) is definitely incompatible with participation in all competitive sports. However, it is important to emphasize that some disease states that produce arrhythmias can be self-limited, with subsequent full recovery.

In general, all athletes with significant cardiac arrhythmias being considered for athletic activity should have a 12-lead ECG, echocardiogram, exercise test and a long-term 24-h Holter ambulatory ECG recording, if possible during the specific type of exercise being considered. Resuscitation equipment and trained personnel may be needed on a standby basis for the latter test, which is deemed important because a conventional exercise test may not replicate the specific clinical situation produced by active participation in the sport. In this regard, exercise tests may need to be adopted specifically for the athletes; that is, to begin exercise at peak energy expenditure, as a sprinter in a race might, rather than with the slow increase in work load commonly used in testing athletes with coronary artery disease.

All athletes with an arrhythmia who are permitted to engage in sports should be reevaluated at intervals after they are "trained" to determine whether the conditioning process affected the arrhythmia. It should also be stressed that athletes with arrhythmias controlled by antiarrhythmic drugs may stop taking these drugs for a variety of reasons, and therefore compliance with recommended therapy must be reestablished periodically. Coaches and team physicians must continually question players about palpitations, with or without physical activity. Abuse with drugs like cocaine can be responsible for life-threatening arrhythmias, and such considerations are an important part of the evaluation.

Specific arrhythmias

DISTURBANCE OF SINUS NODE FUNCTION

Sinus tachycardia and sinus bradycardia that are found to be appropriate for the clinical situation are not considered abnormal. Resting sinus bradycardia is a universal finding in athletes, attributed mainly to enhanced vagal tone. Other proposed mechanisms include reduced sympathetic tone, reduction of both the parasympathetic and sympathetic tone with the major reduction being in the sympathetic tone (20), and independent slowing of the intrinsic rate of the sinus node produced by training (21). Intrinsic heart rate, defined as the heart rate obtained after dual autonomic blockage using propranolol and atropine, was found to be lower in athletes than in controls. Despite the significantly low diurnal and nocturnal variation in athletes in comparison to controls, the pattern of circadian variation is similar in both groups (7, 22). A resting sinus rate below 40 beats/min was seen in about 1.5% of athletes (6, 23), and one study investigating athletes with different levels of training suggested that bradycardia induced by training approaches its lower limit at a moderate level of fitness with only minimal further slowing at a more advanced level of training (7). In general, sinus bradycardia in athletes is considered a physiological phenomenon and requires no specific testing or treatment.

Sinus arrhythmia and wandering pacemaker are generally considered normal and common findings in the young and in athletes, especially with slower heart rates and augmented vagal tone (23). During 24-h continuous electrocardiographic monitoring in 50 male medical students without apparent heart disease, sinus arrhythmia was observed in all of them, and wandering pacemaker was noted at least once in 27 subjects (54%) (24). Athletes with these arrhythmias require no further testing, unless the arrhythmia results in inappropriately slow rates accompanied by symptoms.

Sinus pauses and sinus arrest are disorders of impulse formation with slowing or cessation of the spontaneous sinus nodal automaticity. Sinoatrial exit block is a conduction disturbance, and its differentiation from sinus arrest in the presence of sinus arrhythmia may not be possible without direct recording of the sinus node discharge. Sinus pauses exceeding 2 seconds without second degree atrioventricular block are relatively rare in healthy nonathletes, and have been seen during ambulatory electrocardiographic recording in 0-5% of the healthy population (7, 22, 24, 25). In endurance athletes, sinus pauses greater than 2 seconds are significantly more common than in controls and are found in 13-37% of athletics studied with 24-h Holter monitoring (7, 22, 26), and are less common in teenage athletes (27) than in adult athletes. Although the exact mechanisms predisposing to long sinus pauses in athletes remain uncertain, they are probably related to those responsible for sinus bradycardia. Clinical significance of prolonged ventricular pauses is still controversial. It is difficult to define the critical length of pause at which symptoms develop, because cerebral blood flow depends not only on the interval between heart beats, but also on regional vascular conditions (28-30) and stroke volume, which is known to be increased in athletes (31). The benign nature of pauses up to 3.4 seconds in athletes has been demonstrated in a 3-year follow-up study (26) and appeared to be of no therapeutic or prognostic significance. Sinus pauses up to 12 seconds have been recorded in an asymptomatic veteran athlete (32). The majority of studies in athletes report a maximum pause of 3.0-3.5 seconds. Consequently, it is probably reasonable and safe to consider of no significance asymptomatic sinus pauses or sinoatrial exit block of less than 3 seconds in athletes, with no further workup needed. Symptomatic pauses of more than 3 seconds are abnormal and require careful evaluation including echocardiography to exclude structural heart disease that may co-exist with training-induced arrhythmia, 12-lead ECG and 24-h ECG monitoring and an exercise test. Electrophysiological testing may be necessary, especially in athletes experiencing syncope or near syncope. After careful investigation, permanent pacing may be deemed necessary, especially in athletes with symptomatic pauses or significantly prolonged pauses even if asymptomatic (32) because of possible insidious loss of neural or other bodily function as a result of repeated asystole (33), the possibility of arrhythmia progression and the risk of ventricular fibrillation and sudden death with chronic recurrent prolonged ventricular standstill.

Sick sinus syndrome is a term used to describe a variety of sinus node abnormalities including sinus arrest or exit block, persistent sinus bradycardia of no apparent etiology and inappropriate for the clinical situation, and alternation of paroxysms of atrial tachyarrhythmias and periods of slow atrial and ventricular rates (bradycardia-tachycardia syndrome). Although it can occur in the absence of other cardiac abnormalities, sick sinus syndrome is considered abnormal, and athletes should be evaluated thoroughly for underlying congenital or acquired heart disease. Treatment is usually indicated and generally involves permanent pacemaker implantation (34) alone or in combination with drug therapy to treat the tachycardia in those with tachycardia-bradycardia syndrome.

Recommendations (35)

i) Athletes with presyncope, syncope or other symptoms of arrhythmia must not participate in sports where the likelihood of even momentary loss of consciousness may be hazardous, until the cause of their condition has been determined and treated if necessary.

ii) Athletes with normal or structurally abnormal hearts in whom the bradyarrhythmia is asymptomatic and disappears with activity and in whom bradycardia rate appropriately increases by exercise can participate in all competitive sports. They should be reassessed periodically to determine that training does not aggravate the bradycardia.

iii) Athletes with symptoms such as impaired consciousness and fatigue clearly attributed to the arrhythmia should be treated and if asymptomatic for 6 months during treatment, can participate in all competitive sports after physician reevaluation. They should be reassessed periodically to assure effectiveness of treatment.

iv) Athletes with symptomatic tachycardia-bradycardia syndrome or inappropriate sinus tachycardia should be treated. If asymptomatic for 6 months, they can participate in low intensity competitive sports (class IA) (see classification of sports).

v) Athletes with pacemakers should not engage in sports with a danger of bodily collision because such trauma may damage the pacemaker system.

DISTURBANCES OF ATRIAL RHYTHMS

Premature Atrial Complexes

Premature atrial complexes (PACs) are among the most common arrhythmias in the general population (24, 36-39) and are more often associated with structural heart disease and increase in frequency with age. PACs can be associated with increased vagal activity (40), and administration of atropine can eliminate them in patients with bradycardia (41). This might explain the increased frequency and number of PACs in athletic groups compared to controls (7, 42, 43). Although they can precipitate the occurrence of supraventricular and on rare occasions ventricular tachycardia, PACs are not considered pathological in and of themselves. In the absence of evidence obtained from a careful history and physical examination suggesting the presence of structural heart disease, and in the absence of symptoms other than occasional palpitations, evaluation other than a 12-lead ECG is not necessary.

Recommendations
Athletes with PACs can participate in all competitive sports.

Atrial Flutter (in the Absence of Wolff-Parkinson-White Syndrome)
Atrial flutter is less common than atrial fibrillation in the general population and it is rare in athletes. Paroxysmal atrial flutter can occur in the absence of structural heart disease, while chronic atrial flutter is likely to be associated with underlying heart disease, such as rheumatic or ischemic heart disease, cardiomyopathy, or postoperative cardiac surgery for congenital heart disease. A single stable macroreentrant circuit is known to be the underlying mechanism for atrial flutter. It can be classified, despite some debate on nomenclature, into typical or "common" atrial flutter exhibiting either a counter-clockwise or clockwise rotation around the tricuspid annulus and through a relatively narrow isthmus in the low right atrium bounded anteriorly by the tricuspid valve and posteriorly by the inferior vena cava, and atypical or "uncommon" atrial flutter which is usually more rapid and does not use the low right atrial isthmus (44). The atrial flutter rate is determined by the maximum refractory period within the circuit and is usually 250-350 beats/min for the common form and 350-450 beats/min for the uncommon form. A rapid ventricular response in a 1:1 fashion can occur with slowing of the atrial flutter rate using antiarrhythmic drugs such as class IA and IC, or by enhancing AV conduction with exercise and athletic activity. Atrial flutter with 1:1 ventricular response can cause profound hemodynamic consequences (45, 46), and may be life-threatening, especially during certain activities where the slightest change in mentation imposes a grave risk on the athlete and/or on others.

Although there are suggestions that atrial flutter carries little, if any, thromboembolic risk (47, 48), this risk rises when atrial flutter complicates structural heart disease (49) and chronic anticoagulation may be necessary.

Radiofrequency catheter ablation of the common form of atrial flutter has evolved significantly over the last few years. A better and more sophisticated understanding of the anatomically based macroreentrant circuit (50-56), and the development of new markers for long-term success of the ablative procedure with demonstration of complete bidirectional isthmus block, have led to a cure rate approaching 100% with minimal recurrence rate (44, 57). The uncommon form of atrial flutter does not use the low right atrial isthmus, and is considered a heterogeneous unstable rhythm, frequently degenerating to atrial fibrillation, terminating spontaneously, or stabilizing to common atrial flutter. This type of atrial flutter may be best managed medically.

Because the potential for very rapid ventricular rate exists if the atrial flutter conducts 1:1 to the ventricles (58), electrocardiographic determination of the ventricular response during an exercise test or athletic event during treatment is essential. For some patients with paroxysmal atrial flutter induction of the arrhythmia by atrial stimulation may be necessary before the exercise test. Occasionally, the inducibility of the arrhythmia is only successful during exercise (59). Evaluation should also include an echocardiogram to evaluate for structural heart disease, and a long-term 24-h ECG recording. Electrophysiological study may be indicated in some athletes to determine the type of atrial flutter and for ablation.

Recommendations

i) Athletes with "typical" common atrial flutter should be considered for radiofrequency catheter ablation as the first therapeutic option. After ablation, they can participate in low intensity competitive sports (class IA), and if there is no evidence of arrhythmia recurrence for 4-6 months and in the absence of structural heart disease, participation in all competitive sports should be allowed.

ii) Athletes with medically treated atrial flutter in the absence of structural heart disease who maintain a ventricular rate comparable to that of an appropriate sinus tachycardia during physical activity while receiving therapy can participate in low intensity competitive sports (class IA), with the warning that rapid 1:1 conduction still may occur. However, full participation in all competitive sports should not be allowed unless the athlete has been without atrial flutter for 4-6 months with treatment.

iii) Athletes with atrial flutter and structural heart disease can participate in low intensity competitive sports consistent with the limitations of the heart disease.

iv) Athletes who require anticoagulation should not participate in sports with danger of bodily collision.

Atrial Fibrillation (in the Absence of Wolff-Parkinson-White Syndrome)
Atrial fibrillation is the most frequently encountered arrhythmia in clinical practice, and is associated with a doubling of mortality regardless of the underlying cardiac pathology. Its incidence increases with age, and usually accompanies other disorders such as rheumatic heart disease, mitral valve prolapse, hyperthyroidism, pulmonary emboli and alcoholism. Atrial fibrillation can be paroxysmal or chronic, and in the absence of underlying heart disease or a precipitating factor, it is usually referred to as "lone atrial fibrillation". Symptoms from atrial fibrillation are determined by multiple factors, including the underlying cardiac state, the loss of atrial contraction, and the rate of the ventricular response, which is dependent on the refractory period and conductivity of the atrioventricular node. Atrial fibrillation may result in a decrease in exercise capacity, palpitations, dyspnea and tachycardia-induced myopathy.

Exercise-provoked atrial fibrillation has been only rarely reported (60, 61), but the incidence of atrial fibrillation is increased in competitive athletes (62-66), and is considerably higher than in the general population of the same age. Atrial fibrillation in athletes is not usually related to structural heart disease and is mainly paroxysmal in nature. Some patients appear most susceptible to atrial fibrillation during periods of high vagal tone, whereas atrial fibrillation in others seems more adrenergic dependent.

Atrial fibrillation is thought to be mainly due to multiple circulating random wavelets of leading edge reentry (67). Multiple animal and human studies and clinical observations suggest occasional focal origin of atrial fibrillation due to a single rapidly discharging focus with resultant apparent fibrillatory conduction pattern throughout the atrial mass that fails to conduct on a 1:1 basis (68-72). Atrial fibrillation can also occur in patients with other forms of supraventricular tachycardia such as atrioventricular nodal reentrant tachycardia and atrioventricular tachycardia that are considered intermediary or inciting arrhythmias, with lack of recurrence of atrial fibrillation after successful catheter or surgical ablation of the underlying arrhythmia (73).

It is very important to identify athletes who may have a focal source of atrial fibrillation with potential cure by focal radiofrequency catheter ablation (70, 74). Long-term continuous ECG recording may be helpful.

Atrial fibrillation is associated with an increased risk of stroke and thromboembolic events (75-78) with no difference in stroke risk between patients with paroxysmal and those with persistent chronic atrial fibrillation. Multiple studies have shown the benefit of anticoagulation and antiplatelet therapy in reducing that risk (76, 77, 79-83). Lone atrial fibrillation has a benign nature and prognosis in people under age of 60 with no increased morbidity or mortality (84, 85), and probably has an even more benign prognosis in healthy young athletes.

Treatment of atrial fibrillation can be unsatisfactory, and medical management directed toward controlling the ventricular rate, minimizing embolic risk, and maintaining sinus rhythm, remain the main therapeutical approach. New catheter ablation techniques have been used and are being studied to cure atrial fibrillation (86-88).

Detailed history and physical exam, a 12-lead ECG and an echocardiogram should always be part of the initial evaluation of athletes with atrial fibrillation to search for underlying etiology and to evaluate for structural heart disease. Evaluation should also include determination of the ventricular response in atrial fibrillation during athletic activity or during an exercise test comparable to the intended sports activity. For some athletes with paroxysmal atrial fibrillation, electrical induction of the arrhythmia before the exercise test may be necessary.

Recommendations

i) Athletes with atrial fibrillation in the absence of structural heart disease who maintain a ventricular rate comparable to that of an appropriate sinus tachycardia during physical activity while receiving no therapy or with therapy can participate in all competitive sports.

ii) Athletes who have atrial fibrillation in the presence of structural heart disease who maintain a ventricular rate comparable to that of an appropriate sinus tachycardia during physical activity while receiving no therapy or with therapy can participate in sports consistent with the limitations of the structural heart disease.

iii) Athletes who require anticoagulation should not participate in sports with danger of bodily collision.

Atrial Tachycardia (in the Absence of Wolff-Parkinson-White Syndrome)

Atrial tachycardia is an uncommon form of supraventricular tachycardia and is rare in healthy athletes (24, 89, 90). It is most common in patients with significant structural heart disease. The atrial rate is generally 150-200 beats/min. Atrial tachycardia can be caused by an automatic atrial focus (91-97), or macroreentry. Automatic atrial tachycardia is usually chronic and incessant with a variable response to antiarrhythmic drug therapy, and can evolve to cardiomyopathy even in otherwise healthy young people (98, 99). Macroreentrant atrial tachycardia often develops late after surgery for congenital heart disease (97, 100-103), and the reentry circuit usually exists around a surgical incision, atriotomy scar or anatomical defect. Macroreentrant atrial tachycardia is often difficult to manage and can contribute to mortality in patients with complex heart disease.

Radiofrequency catheter ablation is an excellent therapeutic option for most of the atrial tachycardias. Its effectiveness approaches 90% for automatic focal atrial tachycardia (104), and is about 75% for reentrant atrial tachycardias based on small series of studies (101-103). Athletes with atrial tachycardia should be evaluated with a 12-lead ECG, echocardiogram and long-term 24-h ECG recording. As mentioned for atrial flutter and atrial fibrillation, determination of the ventricular response during an exercise test or an athletic event during medical treatment is also essential. Induction of the atrial arrhythmia by programmed electrical stimulation may be needed in some athletes before the exercise test.

Recommendations

i) Athletes with atrial tachycardia should be first considered for electrophysiologic study and radiofrequency catheter ablation. If there is no evidence of arrhythmia recurrence for 4-6 months after ablation, and in the absence of structural heart disease, participation in all competitive sports should be allowed.

ii) Athletes with atrial tachycardia, in the absence of structural heart disease, who maintain a ventricular rate comparable to that of an appropriate sinus tachycardia during physical activity with or without therapy, can participate in all competitive sports.

iii) Athletes with atrial tachycardia and underlying structural abnormality can participate only in competitive sports consistent with the limitations of the heart disease.

Sinus Node Reentrant Tachycardia (SNRT)

This arrhythmia is another uncommon type of supraventricular tachycardia and is usually slower than the other forms, with an average rate of 130-140 beats/min (105). Patients may be slightly older and have a higher incidence of heart disease than those with supraventricular tachycardia due to other mechanisms. Because of its relatively slow rate, SNRT may not result in serious symptoms. Drug therapy may be effective in terminating and preventing recurrences of SNRT. Catheter or surgical ablation (106-108) to destroy all or part of the sinus node may be necessary with possible need for permanent pacing.

Athletes with SNRT should have a 12-lead ECG, continuous 24-h ECG recording, echocardiogram, and stress testing similar to the evaluation in athletes with atrial tachycardia.

Recommendations

i) Athletes with symptomatic sinus node reentrant tachycardia in the absence of structural heart disease who have no evidence of arrhythmia recurrence 4-6 months after ablation procedure, or who maintain ventricular rate comparable to that of an appropriate sinus tachycardia during physical activity with or without therapy, can participate in all competitive sports.

ii) Athletes with SNRT and underlying heart disease can participate only in competitive sports consistent with the limitations of the heart disease.

iii) Athletes with pacemakers should avoid sports with danger of bodily collision.

Chaotic (Multifocal) Atrial Tachycardia
This arrhythmia is extremely rare in athletes and occurs commonly in older patients with chronic obstructive pulmonary disease and congestive heart failure. Theophylline and to a lesser extent digoxin have been implicated as potential causes. Atrial rates range between 100 and 130 beats/min. Treatment is directed towards the underlying etiology and antiarrhythmic drug therapy is often ineffective.

Evaluation and final recommendations are similar to those for other forms of atrial tachycardias, except that catheter or surgical ablation is not an option.

ATRIOVENTRICULAR JUNCTIONAL RHYTHM DISTURBANCES

Atrioventricular Escape Junctional Beats and Junctional Rhythm
These arrhythmias are common in athletes (23, 109-112) and are considered a result of physical training and vagal hypertonia. AV junctional rhythm was observed in all of the 35 endurance athletes studied by continuous electrocardiographic recording (22). One study suggests that these arrhythmias are less common in teenage athletes than in adult athletes (27). These rhythm disturbances are also observed in healthy nonathletic individuals (24).

Clinical evaluation and recommendations are the same as those for symptomatic athletes with disturbances of sinus node function.

Premature Atrioventricular Junctional Complexes
If the athlete is asymptomatic except for occasional episodes of palpitations that do not suggest a sustained tachycardia, evaluation need include only a 12-lead ECG. In some athletes, a 24-h ECG recording (during athletic activity if possible), echocardiogram and an exercise test may be indicated.

Recommendations
i) Athletes with structurally normal hearts and normal heart rate responses to activity without evidence of sustained tachycardia can participate in all competitive sports.

ii) Athletes with abnormal hearts, can participate in competitive sports consistent with the limitations of the structural cardiac disease.

Nonparoxysmal Atrioventricular Junctional Tachycardia
This arrhythmia occurs most commonly in patients with underlying heart disease or after open-heart surgery (113-115). Available data suggest that nonparoxysmal AV junctional tachycardia is due to abnormal enhanced automaticity. It can cause syncope (116) and other symptoms depending on the rate of the arrhythmia, the underlying etiology and the

severity of the heart disease. Management includes medical therapy, AV junction ablation with permanent pacing (117), and more recently selective ablation of the junctional tachycardia focus, while preserving normal AV conduction (118-121). Because AV block is a significant complication, radiofrequency catheter ablation is recommended only after failure of medical treatment. Junctional tachycardia may be associated with multiple other arrhythmias of focal or reentrant mechanisms (116).

Athletes with nonparoxysmal AV junctional tachycardia should have a 12-lead ECG, echocardiogram, exercise test and 24-h ECG recording during activity.

Recommendations

i) Athletes without structural heart disease who have a controlled ventricular rate that increases and slows appropriately in relation to the level of activity with or without medical therapy can participate in all sports.

ii) Athletes without structural heart disease, who undergo successful radiofrequency catheter ablation with no recurrence of arrhythmia for 4-6 months after ablation, can participate in all sports.

ii) Athletes with pacemakers should avoid participating in sports that involve bodily collision.

iii) Athletes who have structural heart disease or incompletely controlled ventricular rates can engage in low intensity competitive sports (class IA), depending on the nature and extent of the structural heart disease and the ventricular rate.

TACHYCARDIAS INVOLVING THE ATRIOVENTRICULAR JUNCTION

Atrioventricular Nodal Reentrant Tachycardia

Atrioventricular nodal reentrant tachycardia (AVNRT) is the most common form of paroxysmal supraventricular tachycardia in adults (122-124), and accounts for approximately 60% of cases. It commonly occurs in the absence of structural heart disease, and has no particular relationship to a specific form of organic heart disease. AVNRT seems to be more common in women, but it is as common in athletes as in the general population. As in most tachyarrhythmias, symptoms vary depending on the heart rate, the type of physical activity during tachycardia, and the presence or absence of structural heart disease. Syncope can occur as a result of the rapid ventricular rate, or can be related to abnormal vasomotor adaptation to tachycardia. In one study (125), most patients with syncope during tachycardia had an abnormal tilt test, with tachycardia no faster than in patients who had AVNRT without syncope. Syncope can also result from asystole when tachycardia terminates, owing to tachycardia-induced depression of the sinus node automaticity. In the absence of concomitant heart disease, the prognosis is usually excellent.

The rate of AVNRT ranges from 140-240 beats/min and can vary from episode to episode and even within the same long episode, due to the dynamic influence of the autonomic nervous system on both anterograde and retrograde conduction of the AV node. Sometimes enhanced adrenergic tone is needed to initiate and sustain the arrhythmia, and exercise can frequently provoke episodes.

Athletes with AVNRT should be evaluated with a 12-lead ECG, echocardiogram to exclude significant structural heart disease, and a stress test. It is important to identify the rate response of the tachycardia during exercise. If exercise does not induce tachycardia, initiation can be attempted using pacing prior to exercise testing. If the diagnosis of the SVT cannot be made with certainty, and if the clinical therapeutic circumstances warrant it, invasive electrophysiologic study may be indicated.

Radiofrequency catheter ablation therapy has revolutionized the treatment of AVNRT by obviating the need for chronic antiarrhythmic drug therapy or surgical ablation. The overall primary success rate of catheter ablation ranges from 96-100% (126-136). The incidence of inadvertent AV block is less than 1% in large series (137). Although drug therapy is still a reasonable therapeutic option in treating some patients with AVNRT in the general population, because it is curative, radiofrequency catheter ablation is the treatment of choice in athletes.

Recommendations
   i) In the absence of structural heart disease, athletes with asymptomatic nonsustained episodes of AVNRT that are not exercise-induced and do not increase in duration during exercise, can participate in all competitive sports.
   ii) Athletes with symptomatic AVNRT or with reproducible exercise-induced tachycardia should be treated with catheter ablation. If there is no recurrence of tachycardia for 4-6 months after ablation, all competitive sports are permitted.
   iii) After successful catheter ablation, athletes with structural heart disease can participate only in competitive sports consistent with the limitations of the heart disease.

Wolff-Parkinson-White Syndrome and Concealed Bypass Tracts
Paroxysmal supraventricular tachycardia (PSVT) is the most common arrhythmia in patients with accessory atrioventricular pathways (138). Accessory pathways can cause orthodromic atrioventricular reciprocating tachycardia (AVRT) with anterograde conduction down the AV node and retrograde conduction up the accessory pathway (90-95%), or antidromic AVRT with anterograde conduction down the accessory pathway and retrograde conduction up the AV node (5-10%) (139). Orthodromic tachycardia with conduction over a concealed accessory pathway accounts for approximately 30-40% of PSVTs in patients with normal resting ECG. Wolff-Parkinson-White (WPW) pattern is more prevalent in males and has a bimodal age distribution, with peaks during the first year of life and during young adulthood. The majority of adults with ventricular preexcitation have normal hearts, although the association with a variety of acquired and congenital cardiac defects has been reported, including Ebstein's anomaly (140, 141), mitral valve prolapse (142) and cardiomyopathies (143). In patients with concealed accessory pathways, no anterograde conduction over the accessory pathway is possible regardless of the site of the origin of the atrial impulse.

Similar to AVNRT, AVRT can result in significant symptoms related to tachycardia rate, abnormal autonomic vasomotor response during tachycardia (125), and prolonged pause following tachycardia termination (144). More importantly, patients with ventricular preexcitation can be at an increased risk for ventricular fibrillation and sudden cardiac death during atrial fibrillation because of the extremely rapid ventricular response (145) due to conduction over an accessory pathway. This leads to electrical instability and hemodynamic impairment. Cardiac arrest can be the first manifestation of WPW syndrome (146-149). Atrial fibrillation can occur as a primary arrhythmia, or more frequently initiated and preceded by AVRT (73). The combination of atrial fibrillation and AVRT is estimated to occur in 40% of patients (150). Successful bypass tract ablation also eliminates atrial fibrillation in up to 95% of patients (151-154).

In order to be at high risk for sudden cardiac death, patients must have both rapid conduction over the accessory pathway and episodes of atrial fibrillation. Patients with orthodromic AVRT with no apparent ventricular preexcitation on resting 12-lead ECG, may still have unrecognized anterograde conduction over the accessory pathway due to enhanced AV nodal conduction or prolonged intraatrial conduction time with left-sided bypass tracts.

Athletes with WPW electrocardiographic pattern should be evaluated for the risk of sudden death. Features associated with decreased risk include: intermittent preexcitation on 12-lead ECG or ambulatory monitoring (155); sudden loss of ventricular preexcitation during exercise stress testing (156-158); and shortest interval between two ventricular beats conducted over the accessory pathway during atrial fibrillation of more than 300 msec. Features that are associated with relatively increased risk include: history of cardiac arrest due to rapidly conducting atrial fibrillation; a shortest interval between two ventricular beats conducted over the accessory pathway during atrial fibrillation of less than 250 msec; the presence of inducible orthodromic AVRT; and the presence of multiple bypass tracts (159-162).

Up to 20% of asymptomatic patients have the shortest resting rate during induced atrial fibrillation of less than 250 msec (163). The estimated risk of sudden cardiac death in this group is about 0.1% per patient-year (164-166), making the most sensitive indicator of risk (short accessory pathway refractory period) highly nonspecific. Actually, noninvasive testing can help identify those individuals with a low risk of sudden death but does not specify those at high risk.

Evaluation in athletes with WPW pattern should include a 12-lead ECG, exercise test, a 24-h ECG recording during athletic activity, and echocardiogram to exclude associated cardiovascular abnormality. Electrophysiologic study can accurately determine the conduction properties of the accessory pathway, and can provide information about the underlying mechanisms of the clinical SVT which include orthodromic AVRT, AVNRT with or without bystander accessory pathway, and AVRT with multiple bypass tracts.

Over the last few years, catheter ablation has become the first line therapy for symptomatic patients (167-175), with high success rate exceeding 98%, minimal risk of less than 1% (169-175), and approximately 5% of late recurrence of conduction (176, 177). Although extensive noninvasive and invasive testing and catheter ablation of the accessory pathway in asymptomatic patients with ventricular preexcitation are probably not indicated in the general population, they should be seriously considered in athletes, especially those younger than 20 years of age.

Recommendations

i) Athletes with symptomatic AVRT should undergo electrophysiological testing and catheter ablation of the accessory pathway regardless of its conduction properties.

ii) Athletes with AVRT and concealed accessory pathways (documented by appropriate electrophysiological testing) have similar recommendations to those with AVNRT.

iii) Asymptomatic athletes with ventricular preexcitation should be considered for evaluation by electrophysiological testing, and if found to be in the high-risk category for sudden cardiac death, catheter ablation of the accessory pathway should be considered.

iv) Asymptomatic athletes with ventricular preexcitation and shortest resting rates during atrial fibrillation of greater than 250 msec (particularly those older than 20) can participate in all competitive sports. Catheter ablation in this group cannot be justified, especially if the procedure carries more than the ordinary risk of complications due to the location of the accessory pathway.

v) Athletes with successful catheter or surgical ablation can participate in low intensity competitive sports, and if they remain asymptomatic and have no evidence of recurrent accessory pathway conduction for 4-6 months after ablation, can participate in all competitive sports.

vi) Athletes with underlying structural heart disease can participate only in competitive sports consistent with the limitations of the heart disease.

VENTRICULAR RHYTHM DISTURBANCES

Premature Ventricular Complexes

Isolated and even complex forms of ventricular ectopy can occur at times in subjects without identifiable cardiovascular disease. Estimates of the overall incidence range between 10% and 73% (24, 178-182) as assessed by continuous ambulatory ECG recording. The incidence and frequency of ventricular ectopy increase with age (179,182,183). Ventricular ectopic activity was found to be diminished in normal subjects at both extremes of heart rate, namely during sleep (184, 185) and during strenuous exercise (184, 186). Premature ventricular complexes (PVCs) have been related to an increased risk of sudden cardiac death in patients with known ischemic heart disease, myocardial disease (187-191), or decreased left ventricular systolic function (192-194), while they appear to be benign in apparently healthy people with similar long-term prognosis and mortality to those of the healthy general population (195, 196). Multiple studies indicate that ventricular arrhythmias are not any more frequent among trained athletes with healthy hearts than in controls (7, 22, 27, 109, 197-200). According to other studies, physical training favors the occurrence of ventricular ectopy, both during normal daily activities (201, 202) and during exercise (199, 203). Detraining has been associated with decreased frequency and complexity of the ventricular ectopy noted during professional endurance training (204). A longer QTc interval has been described in athletes compared to untrained individuals (201, 202, 205-207). However, no relationship was found between QTc prolongation and severity of ventricular ectopy in athletes. A 5-year follow-up study of endurance athletes with ventricular extrasystoles without evidence of cardiovascular disease, showed an excellent prognosis irrespective of continuing or discontinuing physical training (204). This indicates that the occurrence of ventricular ectopy in otherwise healthy athletes does not seem to be harmful and does not imply an increased risk of sudden cardiac death. Of course the detection of complex forms of ventricular arrhythmias should always prompt careful evaluation in search of underlying cardiac disease.

Exercise and increased sympathetic activity can sometimes suppress ventricular arrhythmias in healthy subjects and increase it in people with organic heart disease (208). However, exercise-induced ventricular ectopy in the absence of apparent cardiac disease has been associated with exercise-induced cardiac arrest (209).

Noninvasive tests recommended for athletes with PVCs include 12-lead ECG, 24-h ECG recording (preferably during athletic activity), echocardiogram and stress test. Even without evidence of structural heart disease, if an increase in the number of PVCs or complex ventricular arrhythmias occurs during exercise, further evaluation is indicated. Signal averaged ECG (SAECG) is another noninvasive test that can be used to improve the identification of arrhythmogenic substrate. The presence of late QRS potentials can help in early detection of patients with coronary (210) or myocardial (211, 212) disease. One recent study (213) of athletes with and without ventricular ectopy showed that ventricular late potentials were only present in athletes with ventricular arrhythmias, and the presence of late potentials correlated with inducible nonsustained ventricular tachycardia during electrophysiological study. Cardiac magnetic resonance imaging, cardiac catheterization and angiography may reveal otherwise undetected abnormalities, including occult coronary artery disease, congenital coronary anomalies, arrhythmogenic right ventricular dysplasia, cardiac tumor or cardiomyopathy.

Recommendations

i) Athletes without structural heart disease (judged by appropriate noninvasive and invasive tests) who have asymptomatic PVCs at rest, during exercise or exercise testing can participate in all competitive sports. Should the PVCs increase in frequency during exercise to the extent that they produce symptoms of impaired consciousness, significant fatigue or dyspnea, the athlete can participate in low intensity competitive sports only (class IA) (see classification of sports).

ii) Athletes with structural heart disease who are in high risk groups and have PVCs (with or without treatment) can participate in low intensity sports only with limitations consistent with the limitations of the heart disease. Athletes with symptomatic PVCs that are suppressed by drug therapy (as assessed by ambulatory ECG recordings) during participation in the sports can compete in low intensity sports only (class IA).

Ventricular Tachycardia

Ventricular tachycardia (VT) is uncommon but not a rare finding in athletes (214). It usually occurs in the presence of cardiovascular disease. It most commonly occurs following myocardial infarction, and can occur with cardiomyopathies and right ventricular dysplasia. Ventricular tachycardia in the absence of identifiable cardiovascular disease is termed "idiopathic".

Sudden death in athletes less than 35 years of age is predominantly due to structural nonatherosclerotic heart disease (215). Ventricular arrhythmias may represent the final common pathways for sudden death in athletes with structural heart disease. Hypertrophic cardiomyopathy is the most common cardiac condition associated with sudden death in young athletes in North America (215), whereas right ventricular dysplasia is the most common potential cause of sudden death in competitive athletes of northern Italy (216). In contrast, sudden death in athletes older than 35 years of age is mostly due to coronary atherosclerosis (217-221).

Ventricular tachycardia that is associated with right ventricular dysplasia usually has left bundle-branch block QRS morphology with left axis and can be fatal (222). Markers of risk for sudden death in right ventricular dysplasia have been suggested (223) and include T-wave inversion in precordial leads; complete right bundle-branch block (RBBB); history of syncope; and spontaneous or induced ventricular tachycardia. Signal averaged ECG (SAECG) shows late QRS potentials in up to 90% of patients with arrhythmogenic right ventricular dysplasia and arrhythmias (139). Magnetic resonance imaging is the most sensitive diagnostic test and is superior to echocardiography, nuclear angiograms, and right ventricular angiography. Reentry seems to be the mechanism of VT in right ventricular dysplasia. Radiofrequency catheter ablation can be successful, making drug treatment a second choice in athletes. Atrial arrhythmias may coexist in up to 24% of patients (224).

Idiopathic VT usually occurs in young patients without underlying structural heart disease, although the presence of an anatomic substrate for idiopathic left ventricular tachycardia has been postulated (225, 226). This VT can be completely asymptomatic, or can be associated with palpitations or syncope. These arrhythmias generally have a good prognosis and are rarely life threatening. SAECG reveals no abnormalities.

The most common idiopathic VT originates from the right ventricular outflow tract (RVOT) (227-231). These tachycardias have a left bundle-branch block (LBBB) pattern with right or left inferior axis. The mechanism appears to be triggered activity, which is promoted by sympathetic stimulation and an increase in intracellular calcium.

Idiopathic VT can also originate from the left ventricle (232-235). In contrast to right ventricular tachycardia, idiopathic left ventricular tachycardia is not usually associated with exertion or stress. It is thought to have a reentrant basis, and usually arises near the inferoposterior septal region of the left ventricle (234, 235). During VT, the QRS complex typically has an RBBB morphology with a superior axis. Radiofrequency catheter ablation is effective in 85-90% of patients with idiopathic VT (104, 227-230, 236) and should be the therapy of first choice in athletes. Calcium channel blockers, beta-blockers and sotalol can also be effective.

Ventricular tachycardia following myocardial infarction is generally caused by relatively large reentry circuit in the old infarct area (237, 238). Pharmacological therapy of this type is often disappointing. Implantable cardioverter defibrillators effectively terminate VT, often with antitachycardia pacing that is well tolerated. Catheter or surgical ablation is still an option in selected patients.

At present, ablation can be considered only for monomorphic ventricular tachycardias, and in most cases, the VT must be well tolerated to allow mapping during the tachycardia.

Evaluation in athletes with ventricular tachycardia should include a 12-lead ECG, exercise test, 24-h ECG recording during exercise, and echocardiography. Cardiac MRI may be needed. Cardiac catheterization is indicated to rule out significant coronary disease or coronary anomaly. Electrophysiological study is also indicated to confirm the diagnosis, and to establish the mechanism of tachycardia and its site of origin.

Recommendations

i) Athletes with nonsustained or sustained ventricular tachycardias should not compete in sports until they are fully evaluated and properly treated with suppression of the ventricular tachycardia.

ii) Athletes with brief episodes of asymptomatic nonsustained monomorphic ventricular tachycardia, rates generally <150 beats/min, and no structural heart disease established by noninvasive and invasive tests, can participate in all competitive sports if exercise testing (preferably by ambulatory ECG recording during the specific competitive sport) demonstrates suppression of the ventricular tachycardia or no significant worsening compared with baseline.

iii) Athletes treated for nonsustained or sustained VT with either ablation or drugs, should not compete in sports for at least 6 months after the last episode of ventricular tachycardia (unless the symptoms produced by tachycardia were very mild, then participation in low intensity competitive sports is permitted during the 6 months after treatment). If there has been no clinical recurrence and VT is not inducible during exercise, exercise testing or electrophysiological study, and the athlete has no structural heart disease, all competitive sports are permitted.

iv) For athletes with structural heart disease and ventricular tachycardia, moderate and high intensity competitive sports are contraindicated regardless of whether the VT is suppressed. Only low intensity competitive sports (class IA) are allowed (see classification of sports).

v) For athletes with an implantable cardioverter defibrillator, all moderate and high intensity sports are contraindicated. The efficacy with which these devices will terminate a potentially lethal arrhythmia under the extreme conditions of competitive sports is currently unknown. These athletes can participate in low intensity competitive sports (class IA) that do not constitute a significant risk of trauma to the device.

Ventricular Fibrillation

Arrhythmic cardiac arrest and sudden cardiac death are the most tragic presentations of cardiac arrhythmias in a trained athlete. Ventricular fibrillation usually occurs in the presence of structural cardiac disease or primary electrical cardiac disorder. It is most commonly associated with coronary artery disease. Ventricular fibrillation due to coronary spasm and myocardial ischemia has been reported in three athletes in the absence of coronary arterial lesions (239). It rarely terminates spontaneously, and death ensues unless counter measures are instituted immediately. Ventricular fibrillation can also occur in relatively young otherwise healthy individuals (idiopathic ventricular fibrillation) (240). In a long-term follow-up study, 13% of patients resuscitated from idiopathic ventricular fibrillation were found to have a family history of unexplained cardiac arrest (241).

In idiopathic ventricular fibrillation, signal averaged ECG is usually normal, as are the QT and QTc intervals (241). Exercise testing can provoke ventricular tachyarrhythmias, but most patients were at rest at the time of ventricular fibrillation. Recurrence of ventricular fibrillation is not infrequent in patients with good left ventricular systolic function and normal coronary arteries, and can occur in up to 37% of patients (241).

An implantable cardioverter defibrillator (ICD) is considered superior to medical therapy, especially if no correctable etiology has been identified (242).

Recommendations

i) Athletes successfully resuscitated from ventricular fibrillation should not compete in sports until they are fully evaluated and properly treated.

ii) Athletes who have had no episode of ventricular fibrillation for 6 months with treatment may engage in low intensity competitive sports only (class IA). Sports that carry a significant risk of trauma to the ICD should be avoided.

Congenital Long QT Interval Syndrome

Patients with congenital long QT syndrome (LQTS) can present with syncope and sudden cardiac death. This syndrome is usually familial with autosomal dominant (243) or autosomal recessive (244) inheritance, but can also be sporadic. Sudden cardiac death is estimated to be the presenting symptom in 9% of pediatric patients with LQTS (245, 246) and reaches 71% in 15 years if untreated (247). The risk of sudden death is increased in those with syncope or with family history of sudden death at a young age. The risk of developing life-threatening ventricular arrhythmias in patients with congenital LQTS is exponentially related to the length of the QT interval corrected for heart rate (QTc). Affected patients may have a normal QT interval that is usually exaggerated during exercise test with abnormal prolongation of the QTc interval at faster heart rates (248). Exercise testing may help to establish the diagnosis, and molecular diagnosis may be useful in some patients.

Patients with LQTS can have ventricular tachycardia (mainly torsade des pointes) which is usually adrenergic-dependent and occurs as a result of exercise, fright or pain. It may also occur during sleep in some patients.

Recent genetic studies showed that congenital LQTS represents a heterogeneous group of patients with abnormalities in sodium or potassium channels related to different genetic abnormalities linked to chromosomes 3, 4, 7, 11 and 21, with more to come in the future (249-252). Augmented sympathetic activity is considered the triggering factor in precipitating ventricular arrhythmias especially in those with abnormal potassium channels, while sleep may be important in those with abnormal sodium channels.

The primary goal of therapy is to prevent sudden cardiac death and life-threatening arrhythmias. Current treatment modalities include beta-blocking agents, left cervicothoracic sympathetic ganglionectomy, and implantable cardioverter defibrillators. Permanent pacing may be added to beta-blocker therapy if associated with pronounced bradycardia. Pacemaker implant may also be indicated to prevent pauses that can be arrhythmogenic with LQTS. Specific genetic therapy may be available in the near future. In patients with congenital LQTS, stressful situations should be avoided and physical overactivity is prohibited even with therapy.

Recommendation

Athletes with congenital LQTS should be restricted from all competitive sports.

ATRIOVENTRICULAR BLOCK

First-Degree Atrioventricular Block

First degree atrioventricular block can occur in healthy individuals (24, 253). It has been reported and is usually more common in athletes evaluated by resting 12-lead ECG or continuous ambulatory electrocardiographic recording (7, 22, 23, 26). It is considered a physiological response to physical training and to increased vagal tone. First degree AV block is more noticeable at rest and during sleep and tends to disappear with activity. Depending on the vagal tone, AV block may normalize or progress to second degree AV block. If the QRS complex on the scalar ECG is normal in contour and duration, the AV delay almost always resides in the AV node, rarely within His bundle, and no further evaluation is necessary. If the QRS complex is abnormal, or the PR interval is excessively prolonged (>0.3 seconds), exercise test, 24-h ECG recording, and echocardiogram are indicated, as well as possibly an electrophysiological study to determine the site and duration of conduction delay.

Recommendations

Athletes with first degree AV block who are asymptomatic, without evidence of structural heart disease, in whom the AV block does not worsen with exercise, can participate in all competitive sports. If underlying heart disease is present, its nature and severity can independently dictate alternative restrictions.

Type I Second-Degree (Wenckebach) Atrioventricular Block

In healthy untrained individuals, second degree AV block tends to occur during sleep, and is rare in the waking state. Chronic second-degree AV block occurs both with and without structural heart disease. In the absence of complicating heart disease, chronic second degree block has a benign prognosis (254, 255), while in the presence of structural heart disease the prognosis is poor and is related to the underlying heart disease. Progression of Wenckebach type I second degree AV block to advanced or complete heart block in adolescents without clinical findings of cardiac disease has been reported (256).

Athletes have increased prevalence of transient Wenckebach block compared to nonathletes (7, 22, 42). The lower prevalence of Wenckebach type I AV block in ex-athletes, and the regression of such AV block on detraining (257, 258), point to the benign nature of this block in healthy athletes. Occurrence of Wenckebach second degree AV block in apparently normal persons, and in trained athletes has been considered a vagally mediated disturbance of impulse conduction localized to the AV node and is regarded as a benign clinical event.

Exercise-induced second degree AV block is uncommon but clinically important because it can result in significant dyspnea or syncope during sports activity, as a result of inappropriate increase or paradoxical decrease in heart rate with exercise. The level of exercise-induced block can be within or distal to His bundle (259-262), but can also occur proximal to His bundle (263).

Recommended tests in athletes with Wenckebach type I AV block include a 12-lead ECG, echocardiogram and exercise test. 24-hour ECG recording during athletic activity may be indicated in some athletes. In those athletes with type I second degree AV block and a coexisting bundle branch block, electrophysiological study may be indicated to identify the presence of His-Purkinje Wenckebach block.

Recommendations

i) Athletes with structurally normal hearts and no worsening or actual improvement of AV block with exercise or recovery can participate in all competitive sports.

ii) Athletes with structurally abnormal hearts in whom AV block disappears or does not worsen with exercise or recovery can participate in all competitive sports, as determined by limitations of the cardiac abnormality.

ii) Athletes without symptoms in whom the AV block initially appears or worsens with exercise or during the recovery period should be evaluated for heart disease and for possible intra- or infra-Hisian block and may require permanent pacing. Such athletes can participate in low intensity competitive sports (class IA).

iii) Athletes treated with pacemakers should not engage in competitive sports with a danger of bodily collision because such trauma may damage the pacemaker system.

Type II Second-Degree Atrioventricular Block

The finding of second degree AV block with Mobitz type II-like pattern is often regarded as indicating a diseased heart. Although a very rare finding in otherwise healthy individuals, type II second degree AV block pattern has been found during ambulatory electrocardiographic recording in competitive athletes (7, 22, 27, 264), with associated narrow QRS complex pointing to the possibility of vagally mediated proximal AV block. Mobitz II-like pattern in athletes represents one of the many situations where differentiation between true type II AV block pattern with infra-Hisian block and a similar pattern with supra-Hisian block can be extremely difficult or even impossible without His bundle recording (265). Exercise-induced infra-Hisian block can occur (259-262).

Evaluation in athletes with this pattern of AV block is similar to that in athletes with Wenckebach type AV block. Electrophysiological study is necessary to verify the level of the block. Permanent pacemaker implant may be needed for treatment.

Recommendations

i) Athletes with type II second degree AV block pattern and block site proximal to His bundle have similar final recommendations to those with Wenckebach type AV block.

ii) Athletes with intra- and infra-Hisian type II second degree AV block should be treated with permanent pacing before any athletic activity, and should not engage in competitive sports with a danger of bodily collision and trauma that might damage the pacemaker system.

Congenital Complete Heart Block

Congenital heart block is the most common cause of AV block in children. Anatomical discontinuity between the atrial musculature and the AV node or the His bundle is a common histological finding. No cause is known for most cases of congenital heart block.

However, it has been associated with connective tissue disease, and various forms of congenital heart disease, the most common being congenitally corrected transposition of the great arteries (266). It is associated with increased morbidity and mortality and can result in syncope (267, 268). Different forms of tachyarrhythmias and bradyarrhythmias have been described to be associated with this type of AV block (269). Broad QRS complex and the presence of associated cardiac defects are considered high-risk markers. The presence of congenital complete heart block does not rule out the ability to perform high levels of physical activity over longer time periods (270-272).

The clinical approach to evaluating the severity of the cardiovascular abnormality includes an echocardiogram, 12-lead ECG, 24-h ECG recording during exercise and exercise stress test (exercise testing should be performed at the same exercise level as that during the sports activity).

Recommendations

i) Athletes with a structurally normal heart and normal cardiac function, no history of syncope or near syncope, a narrow QRS complex, ventricular rates at rest greater than 40-50 beats/min and increases with exercise, no or only occasional premature ventricular complexes and no ventricular tachycardia during exertion can participate in all competitive sports (273).

ii) Athletes with ventricular arrhythmias, symptoms of fatigue, near syncope or syncope should have a pacemaker implanted before they are allowed to participate in competitive sports.

iii) Athletes with pacemakers should not participate in competitive sports with a danger of bodily collision because such trauma may damage the pacemaker system. Before allowing athletes to engage in these activities, an exercise test should be performed at the level of activity demanded by the particular sport to be certain that the paced heart rate increases appropriately.

iv) Athletes with structural heart disease have limitations consistent with the underlying abnormality.

Acquired Complete (Third-Degree) AV Block

Acquired complete AV block occurs most commonly within the bundle of His, or distal to it in the Purkinje system. In the adult, drug toxicity, coronary disease and degenerative processes appear to be the most common causes of complete heart block. Acquired third degree AV block is very rare in athletes, and it can be permanent or transient (274, 275). Of the total 12,000 athletes examined by Fenici *et al.* (276), only two had acquired complete heart block on the resting ECG, and both were asymptomatic. The prognosis of athletes with complete heart block in the absence of underlying heart disease is still uncertain. Its reversibility and benign nature have been suggested by different studies and case reports (257, 276-278). Nevertheless, when a third degree AV block is present, careful clinical evaluation is necessary to exclude the possibility of underlying heart disease. Hypervagotonia is assumed to be responsible for transient complete AV block in some athletes, and deconditioning has been successful in managing symptomatic athletes with third degree AV block (257, 278).

Evaluation of athletes with complete AV block includes 12-lead ECG, echocardiogram, 24-h continuous ECG recording, and exercise test. Electrophysiological study is also indicated to determine the level of AV block.

Recommendations

i) Athletes with structurally normal hearts and asymptomatic transient complete AV block that disappears during exercise with appropriate increase in heart rate, can participate in all competitive sports.

ii) Athletes with symptoms of fatigue, near syncope or syncope should have a pacemaker implanted before they are allowed to participate in competitive sports. Athletes with pacemakers should not participate in competitive sports with a danger of bodily collision because such trauma may damage the pacemaker system. Before allowing athletes to engage in these activities, an exercise test should be performed at the level of activity demanded by the particular sport to be certain that the paced heart rate increases appropriately.

iii) Athletes with structural heart disease have limitations consistent with the underlying abnormality.

ACQUIRED INTRAVENTRICULAR CONDUCTION ABNORMALITIES

Incomplete right bundle-branch block (IRBBB) is the most common intraventricular conduction abnormality noted on the surface ECG in athletes. It is predominantly seen in males (23) and is estimated to occur in about 14% of all athletes (66). IRBBB appears to be related to right ventricular hypertrophy. Its incidence is increased with advanced level of training (257), and it may regress on detraining (279, 280). Complete right bundle-branch block, however, is an infrequent finding in athletes and its incidence is comparable to that of the healthy population (109).

Complete left bundle-branch block is very rare in healthy subjects. It was reported in 0.02% of 21,000 flying personnel studied (65). LBBB is probably more likely than RBBB to be associated with underlying heart disease. Acquired LBBB is rare in children and it is associated with syncope from presumed paroxysmal atrioventricular block.

Acquired complete left or right BBB predicted increased incidence of coronary events or congestive heart failure in a significant number of people according to the Framingham study (281, 282). However, this did not apply to healthy groups where QRS duration failed to predict coronary events in healthy men and women according to a more recent Framingham study report (283).

Exercise-induced BBB is an infrequent entity and can be associated with coronary heart disease (284). The development of permanent LBBB in people with exercise-induced LBBB may be related to underlying coronary or myocardial disease (285).

Athletes with intraventricular conduction abnormality should have a 12-lead ECG, echocardiogram, 24-h continuous ECG monitoring, and exercise test. Invasive electrophysiological study should be considered in symptomatic athletes and in young athletes with complete LBBB.

Recommendations

    i) Asymptomatic athletes with IRBBB and no evidence of underlying heart disease can participate in all competitive sports.

    ii) Athletes with RBBB (with or without left axis deviation) and athletes with LBBB who do not develop AV block with exercise and who have no symptoms can participate in all competitive sports.

    iii) Athletes with a normal HV interval and a normal AV conduction response to pacing, can participate in all competitive sports.

    iv) Athletes with significantly prolonged HV interval (>90 msec) or with a His-Purkinje block should have permanent pacemaker implantation and should be restricted from competitive sports with a danger of bodily collision that might damage the pacemaker system.

    v) Athletes with intraventricular conduction abnormality and structural heart disease can participate in competitive sports consistent within the limitations of the heart disease.

Acknowledgements

This has been supported in part by Herman C. Krannert Fund and by grant HL 52323 from the National Heart Lung and Blood Institute of the National Institutes of Health.

References

1.   Garson, A. Jr., McNamara, D.G. *Sudden death in a pediatric cardiology population, 1958 to 1983: Relation to prior arrhythmias* (abstract). J Am Coll Cardiol 1985, 5 (Suppl. B): 134B.
2.   Vetter, V.L., Edwards, W.D. *Postoperative arrhythmias after surgery for congenital heart defects.* Cardiol Rev 1994, 2: 83.
3.   Driscoll, D.J., Edwards, W.D. *Sudden unexpected death in children and adolescents* (abstract). J Am Coll Cardiol 1985, 5 (Suppl. B): 118B.
4.   Maron, B.J. *Sudden death in young athletes: Lessons from the Hank Gathers affair.* N Engl J Med 329: 55, 1993.
5.   Coumel, P. *Cardiac arrhythmias and the autonomic nervous system.* J Cardiovasc Electrophysiol 1993, 4: 338.
6.   Zehender, M., Meinertz, T., Keul, J., Just, H. *ECG variants and cardiac arrhythmias in athletes: Clinical relevance and prognostic importance.* Am Heart J 1990, 119: 1378.
7.   Bjornstad, H., Storstein, L., Meen, H.D. et al. *Ambulatory electrocardiographic findings in top athletes, athletic students and control subjects.* Cardiology 1994, 84: 42.
8.   Zipes, D.P. *Specific arrhythmias: Diagnosis and treatment.* In: Heart Disease: A Textbook of Cardiovascular Medicine. 5th Ed. Braunwald., E. (Ed.). Saunders: Philadelphia 1997: 640-704.
9.   Ludomirsky, A., Garson, A. Jr. *Supraventricular tachycardia.* In: Pediatric Arrhythmias: Electrophysiology and Pacing. Gillette, P.C., Garson, A. Jr. (Eds.). Saunders: Philadelphia 1990: 380-426.
10.   Muller, J.E., Abela, G.S., Nesto, R.W., Tofler, G.H. *Triggers, acute risk factors and vulnerable plagues: The lexicon of a new frontier.* J Am Coll Cardiol 1994, 23: 908.
11.   DeRose, J.J. Jr., Banas, J.S. Jr., Winters, S.L. *Current perspective on sudden cardiac death in hypertrophic cardiomyopathy.* Prog Cardiovasc Dis 1994, 36: 475.
12.   Stewart, J.T., Mckenna, W.J. *Arrhythmias in hypertrophic cardiomyopathy.* J Cardiovasc Electrophysiol 1991, 2: 516.
13.   Furlanello, F., Bettini, R., Bertoldi, A. et al. *Arrhythmia patterns in athletes with arrhythmogenic right ventricular dysplasia.* Eur Heart J 1989, 10 (Suppl. D): 16.

14. Michael, P.L., Mandagout, O., Vahanian, A. et al. *Ventricular arrhythmias in aortic valve disease before and after aortic valve replacement.* Acta Cardiol 1992, 47: 145.
15. Topaz, O., Edwards, J.E. *Pathologic features of sudden death in children, adolescents, and young adults.* Chest 1985, 87: 476.
16. Vohra, J., Sathe, S., Warren, R. et al. *Malignant ventricular arrhythmias in patients with mitral valve prolapse and mild mitral regurgitation.* PACE 1993, 16: 387.
17. Maron, B.J., Epstein, S.E., Roberts, W.C. *Causes of sudden death in competitive athletes.* J Am Coll Cardiol 19986, 7: 204.
18. Murphy, J.G., Gersh, B.J., Mair, D.D. et al. *Long-term outcome in patients undergoing surgical repair of tetralogy of Fallot.* N Engl J Med 1993, 329: 593.
19. Stevenson, W.G., Stevenson, L.W., Middlekauff, H.R., Saxon, L.A. *Sudden death prevention in patients with advanced ventricular dysfunction.* Circulation 1993, 88: 2953.
20. Badeer, H.S. *The genesis of cardiomegaly in streneous athletic training: A new look.* J Sports Med Phys Fitness 1975, 1: 57.
21. Ordway, G.A., Charles, J.B., Randall, D.C. et al. *Heart rate adaptation to exercise training in cardiac-denervated dogs.* J Appl Physiol 1982, 52: 1586.
22. Viitasalo, M.T., Kala, R., Eisalo, A. *Ambulatory electrocardiographic recording in endurance athletes.* Br Heart J 1982, 47: 213.
23. Bjornstad, H., Storstein, L., Meen, H.D. et al. *Electrocardiographic findings of heart rate and conduction times in athletic students and sedentary control subjects.* Cardiology 1993, 83: 258.
24. Brodsky, M., Wu, D., Denes, P. et al. *Arrhythmias documented by 24 hour continuous electrocardiographic monitoring in 50 male medical students without apparent heart disease.* Am J Cardiol 1977, 39: 390.
25. Bjerregaard, P. *The longest pauses observed during ambulatory electrocardiography in healthy subjects.* Abstracts of the VIIIth European Congress of Cardiology (Paris, 1980): 83.
26. Ogawa, S., Tabata, H., Ohishi, S. et al. *Prognostic significance of long ventricular pauses in athletes.* Japan Circ J 1991, 55: 761.
27. Viitasalo, M.T., Kala, R., Eisalo, A. *Ambulatory electrocardiographic findings in young athletes between 14 and 16 years of age.* Eur Heart J 1984, 5: 2.
28. Wood, J.H. Cerebral Blood Flow. McGrow-Hill Book Co.: New York. 1987: 119.
29. Beil, C. *Comparative analysis of regional brain blood flow and glucose metabolism in focal cerebrovascular disease measured by dynamic positrom emission tomography of fluorine 18-labelled tracers.* J Neurol 1987, 234: 315.
30. Harper, A.M., Deshmukh, V.D., Roman, J.O., Jennett, W-B. *The influence of sympathetic nervous activity on cerebral blood flow.* Arch Neurol 1972, 27: 1.
31. Roeske, V.M., O'Rourke, R.A., Klein, A. et al. *Noninvasive evaluation of ventricular hypertrophy in professional athletes.* Circulation 1976, 53(2): 286.
32. Northcote, R.J., Rankin, A.C., Scullion, R., Logan, W. *Is severe bradycardia in veteran athletes an indication for a permanent pacemaker?.* Br Med J 1989, 298: 231.
33. Guilleminault, C., Pool, P., Moota, J., Gillis, A.M. *Sinus arrest during REM sleep in young adults.* N Engl J Med 1984, 311: 1006.
34. Haywood, G.A., Katritsis, D., Ward, J. et al. *Atrial adaptive rate pacing in sick sinus syndrome: Effects on exercise capacity and arrhythmias.* Br Heart J 1993, 69: 174.
35. Zipes, D.P., Garson, A. Jr. *Task Force VI: Arrhythmias.* J Am Coll Cardiol 1994, 24: 892.
36. Clarke, J.M., Hamer, J., Shelton, JR., et al. *The rhythm of the normal human heart.* Lancet 1976, ii: 509.
37. Hinkle, L.E., Carver, S.T., Stevens, M. *The frequency of asymptomatic disturbances of cardiac rhythm and conduction in middle-aged men.* Am J Cardiol 1969, 24: 629.
38. Scott, O., Williams, G.J., Fiddler, G.I. *Results of 24 hour ambulatory monitoring of electrocardiogram in 131 healthy boys aged 10 to 13 years.* Br Heart J 1980, 44: 304.
39. Sobotka, P.A., Mayer, J.H., Bauernfeind, R.A. et al. *Arrhythmias documented by 24-hour continuous ambulatory electrocardiographic monitoring in young women without apparent heart disease.* Am Heart J 1981, 101: 753.
40. Schuessler, R.B., Boineau, J.P., Bromberg, B.I. et al. *Normal and abnormal activation of the atrium.* In: Cardiac Electrophysiology. From Cell to Bedside. 2nd Ed. Zipes, D.P., Jalife, J. (Eds.). WB Saunders:

Philadelphia 1995: 543-62.

41.   Goel, B.G., Han, J. *Atrial ectopic activity associated with sinus bradycardia.* Circulation 1970, 42: 853.

42.   Talan, D.A., Bauernfeind, R.A., Ashley, W.W. et al. *Twenty-four continuous ECG recordings in long distance runners.* Chest 1982, 82: 19.

43.   Hanne-Paparo, N., Drory, Y., Schoenfeld. et al. *Common ECG changes in athletes.* Cardiology 1976, 61: 267.

44.   Lesh, M.D., Kalman, J.M., Olgin J.E. *An electrophysiologic approach to catheter ablation of atrial flutter and tachycardia: From mechanism to practice.* In: Interventional Electrophysiology. 1st ed. Singer, I. (Ed.). Williams & Wilkins 1997: 347-82.

45.   Robertson, C.E., Miller, H.C. *Extreme tachycardia complicating the use of disopyramide in atrial flutter.* Br Heart J 1980, 44: 602.

46.   London, F., Howell, M. *Atrial flutter: 1 to 1 conduction during treatment with quinidine and digitalis.* Am Heart J 1954, 48: 152.

47.   Arnold, A.Z., Mick, M.J., Mazurek, R.P. et al. *Role of prophylactic anticoagulation for direct current cardioversion in patients with atrial fibrillation or atrial flutter.* J Am Coll Cardiol 1992, 19: 851.

48.   Santiago, D., Warshofsky, M., Giuseppe, L.M. et al. *Left atrial appendage function and thrombus formation in atrial fibrillation-flutter: A transesophageal echocardiographic study.* J Am Coll Cardiol 1994, 24: 159.

49.   Feltes, T.F., Friedman, R.A. *Transesophageal echocardiographic detection of atrial thrombi in patients with non fibrillation atrial tachyarrhythmias and congenital heart disease.* J Am Coll Cardiol 1994, 24: 1365.

50.   Cosio, F.G., Lopez-Gil, M., Goicolea, A. et al. *Radiofrequency ablation of the inferior vena cava-tricuspid valve isthmus in common atrial flutter.* Am J Cardiol 1993, 71: 705.

51.   Cosio, F.G., Goicolea, A., Lopez-Gil, M. et al. *Catheter ablation of atrial flutter circuits.* PACE 1993, 16: 637.

52.   Fischer, B., Haissaguerre, M., Garrigues S. et al. *Radiofrequency catheter ablation of common atrial flutter in 80 patients.* J Am Coll Cardiol 1995, 25: 1365.

53.   Cauchemez, B., Haissaguerre, M., Fischer, B. et al. *Electrophysiological effects of catheter ablation of inferior vena cava-tricuspid annulus isthmus in common atrial flutter.* Circulation 1996, 93: 284.

54.   Poty, H., Saoudi, N., Abdel Aziz, A. et al. *Radiofrequency catheter ablation of type I atrial] flutter: Prediction of late success by electrophysiological criteria.* Circulation 1995, 92: 1389.

55.   Olgin, J.E., Kalman, J.M., Fitzpatrick, A.P. et al. *Role of right atrial endocardial structures as barriers to conduction during human type I atrial flutter. Activation and entrainment mapping guided by intracardiac echocardiography.* Circulation 1995, 92: 1839.

56.   Kalman, J.M., Olgin, J.E., Saxon, L.A. et al. *Activation and entrainment mapping define the tricuspid annulus as the anterior barrier in typical atrial flutter.* Circulation 1996, 94: 398.

57.   Poty, H., Saoudi, N., Nair, M. et al. *Radiofrequency catheter ablation for atrial flutter: Further insights into the various types of isthmus block: Application to ablation during sinus rhythm.* Circulation 1996, 94: 3204.

58.   Garson, A. Jr., Allendet, JH., Baron, P.J. et al. *Atrial flutter in the young: A collaborative study of 380 cases* (abstract). Pediatr Cardiol 1984, 4: 307.

59.   Biffi, A., Ammirati, F., Caselli, G. et al. *Usefulness of transesophageal pacing during exercise for evaluating palpitations in top-level athletes.* Am J Cardiol 1993, 72: 922.

60.   Antman, E.M. *Atrial fibrillation and flutter: Maintaining stability of sinus rhythm versus ventricular rate control.* J Cardiovasc Electrophysiol 1995, 6: 962.

61.   Blackshear, J.L., Safford, R.F., Pearce, LA. *F-amplitude, left atrial appendage velocity, and thromboembolic risk in nonrheumatic atrial fibrillation.* Clin Cardiol 1996, 19: 309.

62.   Chapman, J.H. *Profound sinus bradycardia in the athletic heart syndrome.* J Sports Med Phys Fitness 1982, 22: 45.

63.   Meytes, I., Kaplinsky, E., Yahini, J.H. et al. *Wenckebach A-V block: A frequent feature following heavy physical training.* Am Heart J 1975, 90: 426.

64.   Smith, W.G., Cullen, K.J., Thorburn, I.O. *Electrocardiograms of marathon runners in 1962 Commonwealth games.* Br Heart J 1964, 26: 469.

65. Hiss, R.G., Lamb, L.E. *Electrocardiographic findings in 122,043 individuals*. Circulation 1962, 25: 947.
66. Minamitani, K., Miyagawa, M., Konco, M. et al. *The electrocardiogram of professional cyclists*. In: Sports Cardiology. Lubich, T., Venerando, A. (Eds.). Aulo Gaggi: Bologna 1980, 315
67. Allessie, M., Konings, K., Wijffels, M. *Electrophysiological mechanisms of atrial fibrillation*. In: Atrial Arrhythmias. State of the Art. DiMarco, J.P., Prystowsky, E.N. (Eds). Futura: Armonk 1995: 155-61.
68. Ortiz, J., Igarashi, M., Gonzales, X. et al. *A new, reliable atrial fibrillation model with a clinical counterpart* (abstract). J Am Coll Cardiol 1993, 21: 183A.
69. Ortiz, J., Niwano, S., Abe, H. et al. *Mapping the conversion of atrial flutter to atrial fibrillation and atrial fibrillation to atrial flutter-insights into mechanism*. Circ Res 1994, 74: 882.
70. Haissaguerre, M., Marcus, F.I., Fischer, B. et al. *Radiofrequency catheter ablation in unusual mechanisms of atrial fibrillation: Report of three cases*. J Cardiovasc Electrophysiol 1994, 5: 743.
71. Moe, G.K., Abildskov, J.A. *Atrial fibrillation as a self-sustaining arrhythmia independent of focal discharge*. Am Heart J 1959, 58: 59.
72. Rokas, S., Gaitanidou, S., Moulopoulos, S. *Chronic atrial fibrillation and incessant ventricular tachycardia treated with a single transcatheter ablation*. Int J Cardiol 1991, 33: 437.
73. Klein, G.J., Bashore, T.M., Sellers, T.D. et al. *Ventricular fibrillation in the Wolff-Parkinson-White syndrome*. N Eng J Med 1979, 301: 1080.
74. Jais, P., Haissaguerre, M., Shah, D.C. et al. *A focal source of atrial fibrillation treated by discrete radiofrequency abaltion*. Circulation 1997, 95: 572.
75. Boston Area Anticoagulation Trial for Atrial Fibrillation Investigators. *The effect of low-dose warfarin on the risk of stroke in patients with nonrheumatic atrial fibrillation*. N Engl J Med 1990 323: 1505.
76. Peterson, P., Boysen, G., Godtfredsen, J. et al. *Placebo-controlled, randomized trial of warfarin and aspirin for prevention of thromboembolic complications in chronic atrial fibrillation: The Copenhagen AFASAK study*. Lancet 1989, 1: 175.
77. The Stroke Prevention in Atrial Fibrillation Investigators. *Predictors of thromboembolism in atrial fibrillation. I. Clinical features of patients at risk*. Ann Intern Med 1992, 116: 1.
78. Wolf, P.A., Dawber, T.R., Thomas, H.E. et al. *Epidemiologic assessment of chronic atrial fibrillation and risk of stroke. The Framingham study*. Neurology 1978, 28: 973.
79. *Warfarin versus aspirin for prevention of thromboembolism in atrial fibrillation: Stroke Prevention in Atrial Fibrillation II Study*. Lancet 1994, 343: 687.
80. EAFT (European Atrial Fibrillation Trial) Study Group. *Secondary prevention in nonrheumatic atrial fibrillation after transient ischemic attack or minor stroke*. Lancet 1993, 342: 1255.
81. Ezekowitz, M.D., Bridgers, S,L., James, K.E. et al. *Warfarin in the prevention of stroke associated with nonrheumatic atrial fibrillation*. N Engl J Med 1992, 327: 1406.
82. Connolly SJ., Laupacis A., Gent M. et al. *Canadian atrial fibrillation anti-coagulation (SAFA) study*. J Am Coll Cardiol 1991, 18: 349.
83. The Boston Area Anticoagulation Trial for Atrial Fibrillation Investigators. *The effect of low-dose warfarin in the risk of stroke in patients with nonrheumatic atrial fibrillation*. N Engl J Med 1990, 323: 1505.
84. Kopecky, S.L., Gersh, B.J., McGoon, M.B. et al. *The natural history of lone atrial fibrillation. A population-based study over three decades*. N Engl J Med 1987, 317: 667.
85. Zipes, D.P. *Atrial fibrillation, from cell to bedside*. J Cardiovasc Electrophysiol 1997, 8: 927.
86. Haissaguerre, M., Gencel, L., Fischer, B. et al. *Successful catheter ablation of atrial fibrillation*. J Cardiovasc Electrophysiol 1994, 5: 1045.
87. Swartz, J.F., Pollersels, G., Silvers, J. et al. *A catheter-based curative approach to atrial fibrillation in humans*. Circulation 1994, 90 (Suppl. 1): 1335.
88. Elvan, A., Pride, H.P., Eble, J.N. et al. *Radiofrequency catheter ablation of the atria reduces the inducibility and duration of atrial fibrillation in dogs*. Circulation 1995, 91: 2235.
89. Pantano, J.A., Oriel, R.J. *Prevalence and nature of cardiac arrhythmias in apparently normal well-trained runners*. Am Heart J 1982, 104: 726.
90. Coelho, A., Palileo, E., Ashley, W. et al. *Tachyarrhythmias in young athletes*. J Am Coll Cardiol 1986, 7: 237.
91. Chen, S.A., Chiang, C.E., Yang, C.J. et al. *Sustained atrial tachycardia in adult patients, electrophysiological characteristics, pharmacological response, possible mechanisms, and effects of radiofrequency ablation*. Circulation 1994, 90: 1262.

92. Engelstein, E.D., Lippman, N., Stein, K.M. et al. *Mechanism-specific effects of adenosine on atrial tachycardia.* Circulation 1994, 89: 2645.
93. Tracy, C.M., Swartz, J.F., Fletcher, R.D. et al. *Radiofrequency catheter ablation of ectopic atrial tachycardia using paced activation sequence mapping.* J Am Coll Cardiol 1993, 21: 910.
94. Walsh, E.P., Saul, J.P., Huse, J.E. et al. *Transcatheter ablation of ectopic atrial tachycardia in young patients using radiofrequency current.* Circulation 1992, 86: 1138.
95. Gillette, P.C. *Successful transcatheter ablation of ectopic atrial tachycardia in young patients using radiofrequency current.* Circulation 1992, 86: 1339.
96. Kay, G.N., Chong, F., Epstein, A.E. et al. *Radiofrequency ablation for treatment of primary atrial tachycardias.* J Am Coll Cardiol 1993, 21: 901.
97. Lesh, M.D., Van Hare, G.F., Epstein, L.M. et al. *Radiofrequency catheter ablation of atrial arrhythmias, results and mechanisms.* Circulation 1994, 89: 1074.
98. Gillette, P.C., Smith, R.C., Garson, A. Jr. *Chronic supraventricular tachycardia: A curable cause of congestive cardiomyopathy.* JAMA 1985, 253: 24.
99. Packer, D.L., Bardy, G.H., Worley, S.J. *Tachycardia-induced cardiomyopathy: A reversible form of left ventricular dysfunction.* Am J Cardiol 1986, 57: 563.
100. Lesh, M.D., Kalman, J.M. *To fumble flutter or tackle "tach"? Toward updated classifiers for atrial arrhythmias.* J Cardiovasc Electrophysiol 1996, 7: 460.
101. Van Hare, G.F., Lesh, M.D., Stranger, P. *Radiofrequency catheter ablation of supraventricular arrhythmias in patients with congenital heart disease, results and technical considerations.* J Am Coll Cardiol 1993, 22: 883.
102. Triedman, J.K., Saul, J.P., Weindling, S.N. et al. *Radiofrequency ablation of intra-atrial reentrant tachycardia after surgical palliation of congenital heart disease.* Circulation 1995, 91: 707.
103. Kalman, J.M., Van Hare, G.F., Olgin, J.E. et al. *Ablation of "incisional" reentrant atrial tachycardia complicating surgery for congenital heart disease: Use of entrainment to define a critical isthmus of conduction.* Circulation 1996, 93: 502.
104. Stevenson, W.G., Ellison, K.E., Lefroy, D.C. et al. *Ablation therapy for cardiac arrhythmias.* Am J Cardiol 1997, 80(8A): 56G.
105. Naccarelli, G.V., Shih, H., Jalal, S. *Sinus node reentry and atrial tachycardias.* In: Cardiac Electrophysiology. From Cell to Bedside. 2nd ed. Zipes, D.P., Jalife, J. (Eds.). WB Saunders: Philadelphia., 1994, 607.
106. Sperry, R.E., Ellenbogen, K.A., Wood, M.A. et al. *Radiofrequency catheter ablation of sinus node reentrant tachycardia.* PACE 1993, 16: 2202.
107. Gomes, A., Mehta, D., Langan, M.N. *Sinus node reentrant tachycardia.* PACE 1995, 18: 1045.
108. Sanders, W.E., Sorrentino, R.A., Greenfield, R.A. et al. *Catheter ablation of sinoatrial node reentrant tachycardia.* J Am Coll Cardiol 1994, 23: 926.
109. Bjornstad, H., Storstein, L., Meen, H.D. et al. *Electrocardiographic findings in athletic students and sedentary controls.* Cardiology 1991, 79: 290.
110. Cullen, K.J., Collin, R. *Daily running causing Wenckebach heart-block.* Lancet 1964, 2: 729.
111. Ector, H., Bourgois, J., Verlinden, M. et al. *Bradycardia, ventricular pauses, syncope and sports.* Lancet 1984, 2: 591.
112. Sargin, O.S., Alp, C., Tanci, C. et al. *Wenckebach phenomenon with nodal and ventricular escape in marathone runner.* Chest 1970, 57: 102.
113. Raja, T., Hawker, R.E., Chaikitpinyo, A. et al. *Amiodarone management of junctional ectopic tachycardia after cardiac surgery in children.* Br Heart J 1994, 72: 261.
114. Till, J.A., Ho, S.Y., Rowland, E. *Histopathological findings in three children with His bundle tachycardia occcurring subsequent to cardiac surgery.* Eur Heart J 1992, 13: 709.
115. Braunstein, P.W. Jr., Sade, R.M., Gillette, P.C. *Life-threatening postoperative junctional ectopic tachycardia.* Ann Thorac Surg 1992, 53: 726.
116. Scheinman, M.M., Gonzalez, R.P., Cooper, M.W. et al. *Clinical and electrophysiologic features and role of catheter ablation techniques in adult patients with automatic atrioventricular junctional tachycardia.* Am J Cardiol 1994, 74: 565.
117. Gillette, P.C., Garson, A. Jr., Porter, C.J. et al. *Junctional automatic ectopic atrial tachycardia: New proposed treatment by transcatheter His bundle ablation.* Am Heart J 1983, 106: 619.

118. Hamdan, M., Van Hare, G.F., Fisher, W. et al. *Selective catheter ablation of the tachycardia focus in patients with nonreentrant junctional tachycardia.* Am J Cardiol 1996, 78: 1292.
119. Scheinman, M.M., Gonzalez, R.P., Cooper, M.W. et al. *Clinical and electrophysiologic features and role of catheter ablation techniques in adult patients with automatic atrioventricular junctional tachycardia.* Am J Cardiol 1994, 74: 565.
120. Young, M.L., Mehta, M.B., Martinez, R.M. et al. *Combined alpha-adrenergic blockade and radiofrequency ablation to treat junctional ectopic tachycardia successfully without atrioventricular block.* Am J Cardiol 1993, 71: 883.
121. Ehlert, F.A., Goldberger, J.J., Deal, B.J. et al. *Successful radiofrequency energy ablation of automatic junctional tachycardia preserving normal atrioventricular nodal conduction.* PACE 1993, 16: 54.
122. Josephson, M.E. *Paroxysmal supraventricular tachycardia: An electrophysiologic approach.* Am J Cardiol 1978, 41: 1123.
123. Wu, D., Denes, P., Amat-Y-Leon, F. et al. *Clinical, electrocardiographic and electrophysiologic observations in patients with paroxysmal supraventricular tachycardia.* Am J Cardiol 1978, 41: 1045.
124. Bar, F.W., Brugada, P., Dassen, W.R. et al. *Differential diagnosis of tachycardia with narrow QRS complex (shorter than 0.12 second).* Am J Cardiol 1984, 54: 555.
125. Leitch, J.W., Klein, G.J., Yee, R. et al. *Syncope associated with supraventricular tachycardia: An expression of tachycardia rate or vasomotor response?* Circulation 1992, 37: 680.
126. Mitrani, R.D., Klein, L.S., Hackett, F.K. et al. *Radiofrequency ablation for atrioventricular node reentrant tachycardia: Comparison between fast (anterior) and slow (posterior) pathway ablation.* J Am Coll Cardiol 1993, 21: 432.
127. Chen, S., Chiang, C., Tsang, W. et al. *Selective radiofrequency catheter ablation of fast and slow pathways in 100 patients with atrioventricular nodal reentrant tachycardia.* Am Heart J 1993, 125: 1.
128. Kottkamp, H., Hindricks, G., Willems, S. et al. *An anatomically and electrogram-guided stepwise approach for effective and safe catheter ablation of the fast pathway for elimination of atrioventricular node reentrant tachycardia.* J Am Coll Cardiol 1995, 22: 974.
129. Haissaguerre, M., Gaita, F., Fischer, B. et al. *Elimination of atrioventricular nodal reentrant tachycardia using discrete slow potentials to guide applications of radiofrequency energy.* Circulation 1992, 85: 2162.
130. Jackman, W., Beckman, K., McClelland, J. et al. *Treatment of supraventricular tachycardia due to atrioventricular nodal reentry by radiofrequency catheter ablation of the slow-pathway conduction.* N Engl J Med 1992, 327: 313.
131. Moulton, K., Miller, B., Scott, J. et al. *Radiofrequency catheter ablation for AV nodal reentry: A technique for rapid transection of the slow AV nodal pathway.* PACE 1993, 16: 760.
132. Wu, D., Yeh, S., Wang, C. et al. *A simple technique for selective radiofrequency ablation of the slow pathway in atrioventricular node reentrant tachycardia.* J Am Coll Cardiol 1993, 21: 1612.
133. Kay, G., Epstein, A., Dailey, S. et al. *Role of radiofrequency ablation in the management of supraventricular arrhythmias: Experience in 760 consecutive patients.* J Cardiovasc Electrophysiol 1993, 4: 371.
134. Akhtar, M., Jazayeri, M.R., Sra, J. et al. *Atrioventricular nodal reentry: Clinical, electrophysiological, and therapeutic considerations.* Circulation 1993, 88: 282.
135. Trohman, R.G., Pinski, S.L., Sterba, R. et al. *Evolving concepts in radiofrequency catheter ablation of atrioventricular nodal reentry tachycardia.* Am Heart J 1994, 128: 586.
136. Epstein, L.M., Lesh, M.D., Griffin, JC. et al. *A direct midseptal approach to slow atrioventricular nodal pathway ablation.* PACE 1995, 18: 57.
137. Kalbfleisch, S.J., Morady, F. *Catheter ablation of atrioventricular nodal reentrant tachycardia.* In: Cardiac Electrophysiology: From Cell to Bedside. Zipes, D.P., Jalife, J. (Eds.). WB Saunders: Philadelphia 1995, 1485.
138. Gallagher, J.J., Pritchett, E.L.C., Sealy, W.C. et al. *The preexcitation syndrome.* Pro Cardiovasc Dis 1978, 20: 285.
139. Josephson, M.E., Schibgilla, V.H. *Athletes and arrhythmias: Clinical considerations and perspectives.* Eur Heart J 1996, 17: 498.
140. Smith, W.M., Gallagher, J.J., Kerr, C.R. et al. *The electrophysiologic basis and management of symptomatic recurrent tachycardia in patients with Ebstein's anomaly of the tricuspid valve.* Am J Cardiol 1982,

49: 1223.

141. Rossi, L., Thiene, S. *Mild Ebstein's anomaly associated with supraventricular tachycardia and sudden death; clinicomorphologic features in 3 patients.* Am J Cardiol 1984, 53: 332.

142. Rechavia, E., Mager, A., Birnbaum, Y. et al. *Mitral valve prolapse, sick sinus and Wolff-Parkinson-White syndromes: Interrelationships with respect to sudden cardiac death.* Isr J Med Sci 1993, 29: 654.

143. Krikler, D.M., Davies, M.J., Rowland, E. et al. *Sudden death in hypertrophic cardiomyopathy: Associated accessory atrioventricular pathways.* Br Heart J 1980, 43: 245.

144. Miller, J.M. *Therapy of Wolff-Parkinson-White syndrome and concealed bypass tracts.* J Cardiovasc Electrophysiol 1996, 7: 85.

145. Dreifus, L.S., Haiat, R., Watanabe, Y. et al. *Ventricular fibrillation: A possible mechanism of death in patients with Wolff-Parkinson-White syndrome.* Circulation 1971, 43: 520.

146. Berkman, N.L., Lamb, L.E. *The Wolff-Parkinson-White syndrome electrocardiogram: A follow up study of 5 to 28 years.* N Engl J Med 1968, 278: 492.

147. Smith, R.F. *The Wolff-Parkinson-White syndrome as an aviation risk.* Circulation 1964, 29: 672.

148. Milstein, S., Sharma, A.D., Klein, G.J. *Electrophysiologic profile of asymptomatic Wolff-Parkinson-White pattern.* Am J Cardiol 1986, 57: 1097.

149. Montoya, P.J. and the European Registry on Sudden Death in Wolff-Parkinson-White syndrome. *Ventricular fibrillation in the Wolff-Parkinson-White syndrome.* Circulation 1988, 78 (Suppl. II): 88.

150. Josephson, M.E. *Clinical cardiac electrophysiology.* Lea & Febiger: Pennsylvania 1993, 343.

151. Sharma, A.D., Klein, G.J., Guiraudon, G.M. et al. *Atrial fibrillation in patients with Wolff-Parkinson-White syndrome: Incidence after surgical ablation of the accessory pathway.* Circulation 1985, 72: 161.

152. Haissaguerre, M., Fischer, B., Labbe, T. et al. *Frequency of recurrent atrial fibrillation after catheter ablation of overt accessory pathways.* Am J Cardiol 1992, 69: 493.

153. Chen, P.S., Pressley, J.C., Tang, A.S.L. et al. *New observations on atrial fibrillation before and after surgical treatment in patients with the Wolff-Parkinson-White syndrome.* J Am Coll Cardiol 1992, 19: 974.

154. Kalbfleisch, S.J., El-Atassi, R., Calkins, H. et al. *Inducibility of atrial fibrillation before and after radiofrequency catheter ablation of accessory atrioventricular connections.* J Cardiovasc Electrophysiol 1993, 4: 499.

155. Klein, G.J., Gulamhusein, S.S. *Intermittent preexcitation in the Wolff-Parkinson-White syndrome.* Am J Cardiol 1983, 52: 292.

156. Strasberg, B., Ashley, W.W., Wyndham, C.R.C. et al. *Treadmill exercise testing in the Wolff-Parkinson-White syndrome.* Am J Cardiol 1980, 45: 742.

157. Eshchar, Y., Belhassen, B., Laniad, S. *Comparison of exercise and ajmaline tests with electrophysiologic study in the Wolff-Parkinson-White syndrome.* Am J Cardiol 1986, 57: 782.

158. Sharma, A.D., Yee, R., Guiraudon, G. et al. *Sensitivity and specificity of invasive and noninvasive testing for risk of sudden death in Wolff-Parkinson-White syndrome.* J Am Coll Cardiol 1987, 10: 373.

159. Tomer Montoya, P.T., Brugada, P., Smeets, J. et al. *Ventricular fibrillation in the Wolff-Parkinson-White syndrome.* Eur Heart J 1991, 12: 144.

160. Bauernfeind, R.A., Wyndham, C.R., Swiryn, S.P. et al. *Paroxysmal atrial fibrillation in the Wolff-Parkinson-White syndrome.* Am J Cardiol 1981, 47: 562.

161. Teo, W.S., Klein, G.J., Guiraudon, G.M. et al. *Multiple accessory pathways in the Wolff-Parkinson-White syndrome as a risk factor for ventricular fibrillation.* Am J Cardiol 1991, 67: 889.

162. Attoyan, C., Haissaguerre, M., Dartigues, J.F. et al. *Ventricular fibrillation in Wolff-Parkinson-White syndrome: Predictive factors.* Arch Mal Coeur Vaiss 1994, 87: 889.

163. Leitch, J.W., Klein, G.J., Yee, R. et al. *Prognostic value of electrophysiologic testing in asymptomatic patients with Wolff-Parkinson-White pattern.* Circulation 1990, 82: 1718.

164. Munger, T.M., Packer, D.L., Hammill, S.C. et al. *A population study of the natural history of Wolff-Parkinson-White syndrome in Olmsted County, Minnesota, 1953-1989.* Circulation 1993, 87: 866.

165. Berkman, N.L., Lamb, L.E. *The Wolff-Parkinson-White electrocardiogram: A follow up study of five to twenty-eight years.* N Engl J Med 1968, 278: 492.

166. Guize, L., Soria, R., Chaouat, J.C. et al. *Prevalence and natural history of Wolff-Parkinson-White syndrome in a population of 138,048 people.* Ann Inter Med 1985, 136: 474.

167. Jackman, W.M., Wang, X., Friday, K.J. et al. *Catheter ablation of accessory atrioventricular pathways (Wolff-Parkinson-White syndrome) by radiofrequency current.* N Engl J Med 1991, 324: 1605.

168. Jackman, W.M., Friday, K.J., Yeung-Lai-Wah, et al. *New catheter technique for recording left free-wall accessory atrioventricular pathway activation: Identification of pathway fiber orientation.* Circulation 1988, 78: 598.

169. Kay, G.N., Epstein, A.E., Dailey, S.M. et al. *Role of radiofrequency ablation in the management of supraventricular arrhythmias: Experience in 760 consecutive patients.* J Cardiovasc Electrophysiol 1993, 4: 371.

170. Kuck, K.H., Schluter, M. *Single-catheter approach to radiofrequency current ablation of left-sided accessory pathways in patients with Wolff-Parkinson-White syndrome.* Circulation 1991, 84: 2366.

171. Calkins, H., Langberg, J., Sousa, J. et al. *Radiofrequency catheter ablation of accessory atrioventricular connections in 250 patients.* Circulation 1992, 85: 1337.

172. Swartz, J.F., Tracy, C.M., Fletcher, R.D. *Radiofrequency endocardial catheter ablation of accessory atrioventricular pathway atrial insertion sites.* Circulation 1993, 87: 487.

173. Lesh, M.D., Van Hare, G.F., Scheinman, M.M. et al. *Comparison of the retrograde and transseptal methods for ablation of left free wall accessory pathways.* J Am Coll Cardiol 1993, 22: 542.

174. Cappato, R., Schluter, M., Mont, L. et al. *Anatomic, electrical, and mechanical factors affecting bipolar endocardial elctrograms: Impact on catheter ablation of manifest left free-wall accessory pathways.* Circulation 1994, 90: 884.

175. Haissaguerre, M., Marcus, F., Poquet, F. et al. *Electrocardiographic characteristics and catheter ablation of parahissian accessory pathways.* Circulation 1994, 90: 1124.

176. Langberg, J.J., Calkins, H., Kim, Y.N. et al. *Recurrence of conduction in accessory atrioventricular connections after initially successful radiofrequency catheter ablation.* J Am Coll Cardio 1992, 119: 1588.

177. Chen, X., Kottkamp, H., Hindricks, G. et al. *Recurrence and late block of accessory pathway conduction following radiofrequency catheter ablation.* J Cardiovasc Electrophysiol 1994, 5: 650.

178. De Maria, A.N., Amsterdam, E.A., Vismara, L.A. et al. *Arrhythmias in the mitral valve prolapse syndrome: Prevalence, nature and frequency.* Ann Intern Med 1976, 84: 656.

179. Raftery, E.B., Cashman, B.M.M. *Long-term recording of the electrocardiogram in a normal population.* Postgr Med J 1976, 52 (Suppl. 7): 32.

180. Clarke, J.M., Hamer, J., Shelton, J.R. et al. *The rhythm of the normal human heart.* Lancet 1976, 2: 508.

181. Bjerrgaard, P. *Prevalence and variability of cardiac arrhythmias in healthy subjects.* In: Cardiac Arrhythmias in the Active Population. Chamberlain, D.A., Kulbertus, H., Morgensen, L., Schlepper, M. (Eds.).: A Lindgren & Soner: Molndal 1980, 24-32.

182. Kostis, J.B., McCrone, K., Moreyra, A.E. et al. *Premature ventricular complexes in the absence of identifiable heart disease.* Circulation 1981, 63: 1351.

183. Hinkle, L.E., Carver, S.J., Argyros, D.C. *The prognostic significance of ventricular premature contractions in healthy people and in people with coronary heart disease.* Acta Cardiol 1974, (Suppl.) 18: 5.

184. Pickering, T.G., Johnston, J., Honour, A.J. *Comparison of the effects of sleep, exercise and autonomic drugs on ventricular extrasystoles, using ambulatory monitoring of electrocardiogram and electroencephalogram.* Am J Med 1978, 65: 575.

185. Winkle, R.A. *The relationship between ventricular ectopic beat frequency and heart rate.* Circulation 1982, 66: 439.

186. McHenry, P.L., Morris, S.N., Kavalier, M. et al. *Comparative study of exercise-induced ventricular arrhythmias in normal subjects and patients with documented coronary artery disease.* Am J Cardiol 1976, 37: 609.

187. Chiang, B.N., Pearlman, L.V., Ostrander, I.D Jr. et al. *Relationship of premature ventricular systoles to coronary heart disease and to sudden cardiac death in Tecumseh Epidemiologic Study.* Ann Intern Med 1969, 70: 1159.

188. Coronary Drug Research Project Group. *Prognostic importance of premature beats following myocardial infarction: Experience in the coronary drug project.* J Am Med Ass 1973, 223: 1116.

189. Ruberman, W., Weinblatt, E., Goldberg, J.D. et al. *Ventricular premature beats and mortality after myocardial infarction.* N Engl J Med 1977, 297: 750.

190. Moss, A.J. *Clinical significance of ventricular arrhythmia in patients with and without coronary artery disease.* Prog Cardiovasc Dis 1980, 23: 33.

191. Bigger, J.T. *Definition of benign versus malignant ventricular arrhythmias: Targets for treatment.* Am J Cardiol 1982, 52: 47C.

192. Schulze, R.A. Jr., Strauss, H.W., Pitt, B. *Sudden death in the year following myocardial infarction: Relation to ventricular premature contractions in the late hospital phase and left ventricular ejection fraction.* Am J Med 1977, 62: 192.

193. Califf, R.M., McKinnis, R.A., Burks, J. et al. *Prognostic implications of ventricular arrhythmias during 24 hour ambulatory monitoring in patients undergoing cardiac catheterization for coronary artery disease.* Am J Cardiol 1982, 50: 23.

194. Multicenter Postinfarction Research Group. *Risk stratification and survival after myocardial infarction.* N Engl J Med 1983, 309: 331.

195. Kennedy, H.L., Underhill, S. *Frequent and complex ventricular ectopy in apparently healthy subjects.* Am J Cardiol 1976, 38: 141.

196. Kennedy, H.L., Whitlock, J.A., Sprague, M.K. et al. *Long-term follow-up of asymptomatic healthy subjects with frequent and complex ventricular ectopy.* N Engl J Med 1985, 312: 193.

197. Hanne-Paparo, N., Kellermann, J.J. *Long-term Holter ECG monitoring of athletes.* Med Sci Sports Exerc 1981, 13: 294.

198. Vitasalo, M.T., Kala, R., Eisalo, A. *Ambulatory electrocardiographic recording in endurance athletes.* Br Heart J 1982, 47: 213.

199. Northcote, R., MacFarlane, P., Ballantyne, D. *Ambulatory electrocardiography in squash players.* Br Heart J 1983, 50: 372.

200. Pilcher, G.F., Cook, A-J., Johnston, B.L. et al. *Twenty four hours continuous electrocardiography during exercise and free activity in 80 apparently healthy runners.* Am J Cardiol 1983, 52: 859.

201. Palatini, P., Maraglino, G., Calzavara, A. et al. *Prevalence and possible mechanism of ventricular arrhythmias in athletes.* Am Heart J 1985, 110: 560.

202. Palatini, P., Maraglino, G., Mos, L. et al. *Effect of endurance training on Q-T interval and cardiac electrical stability in boys aged 10 to 14.* Cardiology 1987, 74: 400.

203. Pantano, J., Oriel, R. *Prevalence and nature of cardiac arrhythmias in apparently normal well-trained runners.* Am Heart J 1982, 104: 762.

204. Palatini, P., Scanavacca, G., Bongiovi, S. et al. *Prognostic significance of ventricular extrasystoles in healthy professional athletes: Results of a 5-year follow-up.* Cardiology 1993, 82: 286.

205. Jordaens, L., Missault, L., Pelleman, G. et al. *Comparison of athletes with life-threatening ventricular arrhythmias with two groups of healthy athletes and a group of normal control subjects.* Am J Cardiol 1994, 74: 1124.

206. Van Ganse, W., Versee, L., Eilenbosch, W. et al. *The electrocardiogram of athletes. Comparison with untrained subjects.* Br Heart J 1970, 32: 160.

207. Hanne Paparo, N., Drory, Y., Schaenfeld, Y. et al. *Common ECG changes in athletes.* Cardiology 1976, 61: 267.

208. Lombardi, F., Malfatto, G., Belloni, A. et al. *Effects of sympathetic activation on ventricular ectopic beats in subjects with and without evidence of organic heart disease.* Eur Heart J 1987, 8: 1065.

209. Cantwell, J.D. *The athlete's heart syndrome.* Int J Cardiol 1987, 17: 1.

210. Solomon, A.J., Tracy, C.M. *The signal-averaged electrocardiogram in predicting coronary artery disease.* Am Heart J 1991, 122: 1334.

211. Vacek, J.L., Scott Smith, G. *The effects of exercise during viremia on the signal-averaged electrocardiogram.* Am Heart J 1972, 119: 702.

212. Mehta, D., McKenna, W.J., Ward, D.E. et al. *Significance of signal-averaged electrocardiography in relation to endomyocardial biopsy and ventricular stimulation studies in patients with ventricular tachycardia without clinically apparent heart disease.* J Am Coll Cardiol 1989, 14: 372.

213. Biffi, A., Ansalone, G., Verdile L. et al. *Ventricular arrhythmias and athlete's heart.* Eur Heart J 1996, 17: 557.

214. Biffi, A., Pelliccia, A., Caselli, G. *Arrhythmias in athletes.* Am Heart J 1986, 112: 1349.

215. Opie, L.H. *Sudden death and sport.* Lancet 1975, 1: 263.

216. Corrado, D., Thiene, G., Nava, A., Rossi, L., Pennelli, N. *Sudden cardiac death in young competitive athletes: Clinicopathologic correlation in 22 cases.* Am J Med 1990, 89: 588.

217. Maron, B.J., Epstein, S.E., Roberts, W.C. *Causes of sudden death in competitive athletes.* J Am Coll Cardiol 1986, 7: 204.

218. Waller, B.F., Roberts, W.C. *Sudden death while running in conditioned runners aged 40 years or over.* Am J Cardiol 1980, 45: 1292.
219. Hawley, D.A., Slentz, K., Clarke, M.A. et al. *Athletic fatalities.* Am J Forensic Med Pathol 1990, 11: 124.
220. Virmani, I.R., Rabinowitz, M., McAllister, H.A. *Nontraumatic death in joggers: A series of 30 patients at autopsy.* Am J Med 1982, 72: 874.
221. Northcote, R.J., Evans, A.D.B., Ballantyne, D. *Sudden death in squash players.* Lancet 1984, 1: 148.
222. Marcus, F.I., Fontaine, G. *Arrhythmogenic right ventricular dysplasia/cardiomyopathy: A review.* PACE 1995, 18: 1298.
223. Furlanello, F., Bettini, R., Bertoldi, A. et al. *Arrhythmia patterns in athletes with arrhythmogenic right ventricular dysplasia.* Eur Heart J 1989, 10 (Suppl. D): 16.
224. Tonet, J., Castro, M.R., Iwa, T. et al. *Frequency of supraventricular tachyarrhythmias in arrhythmogenic right ventricular dysplasia.* Am J Cardiol 1991, 67: 1153.
225. Thakur, R., Klein, G.J., Sivaram, C.A. et al. *Anatomic substrate for idiopathic left ventricular tachycardia.* Circulation 1996, 93: 497.
226. Suwa, M., Yoneda, Y., Nagao, H. et al. *Surgical correction of idiopathic paroxysmal ventricular tachycardia possibly related to left ventricular false tendon.* Am J Cardiol 1989, 64: 1217.
227. Klein, L.S., Shih, H.-T., Hackett, K. et al. *Radiofrequency catheter ablation of ventricular tachycardia in patients without structural heart disease.* Circulation 1992, 85: 1666.
228. Coggins, D.L., Lee, R.J., Sweeney, J. et al. *Radiofrequency catheter ablation as a cure for idiopathic tachycardia of both left and right ventricular origin.* J Am College Cardiol 1994, 23: 1333.
229. Calkins, H., Kalbfleisch, S.J., El-Atassi, R. et al. *Relation between efficacy of radiofrequency catheter ablation and site of origin of idiopathic ventricular tachycardia.* Am J Cardiol 1993, 71: 827.
230. Wilber, D.J., Baerman, J., Olshansky, B. et al. *Adenosine-sensitive ventricular tachycardia.* Circulation 1993, 87: 126.
231. Lerman, B., Stein, K., Engelstein, E.D. et al. *Mechanism of repetitive monomorphic ventricular tachycardia.* Circulation 1995, 92: 421.
232. Belhassen, B., Viskin, S. *Idiopathic ventricular tachycardia and ventricular fibrillation.* J Cardiovasc Electrophysiol 1993, 4: 356.
233. Ohe, T., Aihara, N., Kamakura, S. et al. *Long-term outcome of verapamil-sensitive ventricular tachycardia in patients without structural heart disease.* J Am Coll Cardiol 1995, 25: 54.
234. Nakagawa, H., Beckman, K.J., McClelland, J.H. et al. *Radiofrequency catheter ablation of idiopathic left ventricular tachycardia guided by a Purkinje potential.* Circulation 1993, 88: 2607.
235. Wen, M.-S., Yeh, S.-J., Wang, C.-C. et al. *Radiofrequency catheter ablation therapy in idiopathic left ventricular tachycardia with no obvious structural heart disease.* Circulation 1994, 89: 1690.
236. Mont, L., Siexas, T., Brugada, J. et al. *The electrocardiographic, clinical, and electrophysiologic spectrum of idiopathic monomorphic ventricular tachycardia.* Am Heart J 1992, 124: 746.
237. Stevenson, W.G., Weiss, J.N., Wiener, I. et al. *Slow conduction in the infarct scar: Relevance to the occurrence, detection, and ablation of ventricular reentry circuits resulting from myocardial infarction.* Am Heart J 1989, 117: 452.
238. Pogwizd, S.M., Hoyt, R.H., Saffitz, J.E. et al. *Reentrant and focal mechanisms underlying ventricular tachycardia in the human heart.* Circulation 1992, 86: 1872.
239. Buja, G., Meneghello, M.P., Belletto, F. *Isolated episode of exercise-related ventricular fibrillation in a healthy athlete.* Int J Cardiol 1989, 24: 121.
240. Meissner, M.D., Lehmann, N.M., Steiman, R.T. et al. *Ventricular fibrillation in patients without significant structural heart disease: A multicenter experience with implantable cardioverter defibrillator therapy.* J Am Coll Cardiol 1993, 21: 1406.
241. Wever, E.F.D., Hauer, R.N.W., Oomen, A. et al. *Unfavorable outcome in patients with primary electrical disease who survived an episode of ventricular fibrillation.* Circulation 1993, 88: 1021.
242. The Antiarrhythmics versus Implantable Defibrillators (AVID) investigators. *A comparison of antiarrhythmic-drug therapy with implantable defibrillator in patients resuscitated from near-fatal ventricular arrhythmias.* N Engl J Med 1997, 337(22): 1621.
243. Ward, O.C. *A new familial cardiac syndrome in children.* J Irish Med Assoc 1964, 54: 103.
244. Jervell, A., Lange-Nielson, F. *Congenital deafness: Functional heart disease with prolongation of the QT interval and sudden death.* Am Heart J 1957, 54: 59.

245. Villain, E., Levy, M., Kachaner, J. et al. *Prolonged QT interval in neonates: Benign, transient, or prolonged risk of sudden death.* Am Heart J 1992, 124: 194.
246. Garson, A. Jr., Dick, M. II, Fournier, A. et al. *The long QT syndrome in children: An international study of 287 patients.* Circulation 1993, 87: 1866.
247. Schwartz, P.J. *Idiopathic long QT syndrome: Progress and questions.* Am Heart J 1985, 109: 339.
248. Vincent, G.M., Jaiswal, D., Timothy, K.W. *Effects of exercise on heart rate, QT, Qtc and QT/QS2 in the Romano-Ward inherited long QT syndrome.* Am J Cardiol 1991, 68: 498.
249. Priori, S.G., Napolitano, C., Paganini, V. et al. *Molecular biology of the long QT syndrome: Impact on management.* PACE 20 (Part II): 2052.
250. Curran, M.E., Splawski, I., Timothy, K.W. et al. *A molecular basis for cardiac arrhythmia: HERG mutations cause long QT syndrome.* Cell 1995, 80: 795.
251. Wang, Q., Shen, J., Splawski, I. et al. *SCN5A mutations associated with an inherited cardiac arrhythmia, long QT syndrome.* Cell 1995, 80: 805.
252. Watig, Q., Curran, M.E., Splawski, I. et al. *Positional cloning of a novel potassium channel gene: KvLQT1 mutations cause cardiac arrhythmias.* Nature Genet 1996, 12: 17.
253. Southall, D.P., Johnston, F., Shinebourne, E.A., Johnston, P.G.B. *24-hour electrocardiographic study of heart rate and rhythm patterns in population of healthy children.* Br Heart J 1981, 45: 281.
254. Strasberg, B., Amat-Y-Leon, F., Dhingra, RC. et al. *Natural history of chronic second-degree atrioventricular nodal block.* Circulation 1981, 63(5): 1043.
255. Hanne-Paparo, N. *Long-term ECG monitoring of a sportsman with second degree A-V block.* Sports Cardiology Bologna, Aulo Gaggi 1980, 559.
256. Young, D., Eisenberg, R., Fish, B., Fisher, J.D. *Wenckebach atrioventricular block (Mobitz I) in children and adolescents.* Am J Cardiol 1977, 40: 393.
257. DiNardo-Ekery, D., Abedin, Z. *High degree atrioventricular block in a marathoner with 5-year follow-up.* Am Heart J 1987, 113: 834.
258. Murayama, M., Kuroda, Y. *Cardiovascular future of athletes.* Sports Cardiol Bologna, Aulo Gaggi 1980, 401-13.
259. Woelfel, A.K., Simpson, R.J., Gettes, L.S., Foster, J.R. *Exercise-induced distal atrioventricular block.* J Am Coll Cardiol 1983, 2: 578.
260. Freeman, G., Hwang, M.H., Danoviz, J., Moran, J.F., Gunnar, R.M. *Exercise induced "Mobitz type III" second degree AV block in a patient with chronic bifascicular block (right bundle branch block and left anterior hemiblock).* J Electrocardiol 1984, 17: 409.
261. Peller, O.G., Moses, J.W., Kligfield, P. *Exercise-induced atrioventricular block: Report of three cases.* Am Heart J 1988, 115: 1315.
262. Chokshi, S.K., Sarmiento, J., Nazari, J. et al. *Exercise-provoked distal atrioventricular block.* Am J Cardiol 1990, 66: 114.
263. Sumiyoshi, M., Nakata, Y., Yasuda, M. et al. *Clinical and electrophysiologic features of exercise-induced atrioventricular block.* Am Heart J 1996, 132: 1277.
264. Kala, R., Viitasalo, M.T. *Atrioventricular block, including Mobitz type II-like pattern, during ambulatory ECG recording in young athletes aged 14 to 16 years.* Ann Clin Res 1982, 14: 53.
265. Zipes, D.P. *Second-degree atrioventricular block.* Circulation 1979, 60: 465.
266. Michaelsson, M. *Congenital complete atrioventricular block.* Progr Pediatr Cardiol 1995, 4: 1.
267. Molthan, M.E., Miller, R.A., Hastreiter, A.R., Paul, M.H. *Congenital heart block with fatal Adams-Stokes attacks in childhood.* Pediatr 1962, 30: 32.
268. Michaellson, M., Engle, M.A. *Congenital complete heart block: An international study of the natural history.* Cardiovasc Clin 1972, 4: 86.
269. Levy, A.M., Camm, A.J., Keane, J.F. *Multiple arrhythmias detected during nocturnal monitoring in patients with congenital complete heart block.* Circulation 1977, 55(2): 247.
270. Paul, M.H., Rudolph, A.M., Nadas, A.S. *Congenital complete atrioventricular block: Problems of clinical assessment.* Circulation 1958, 18: 183.
271. Thoren, C., Herin, P., Vavra, J. *Studies of submaximal and maximal exercise in congenital complete heart block.* Acta Paediatr Belg 1974, 28: 132.
272. Winkler, R.B., Freed, M., Nadas, A. *Exercise-induced ventricular ectopy in children and young adults with complete heart block.* Am Heart J 1980, 99: 87.

273. Karpawich, P.P., Gillette, P.C., Garson, A. Jr. et al. *Congenital complete atrioventricular block: Clinical and electrophysiologic predictors of need for pacemaker insertion.* Am J Cardiol 1981, 48: 1098.
274. Wolffe, J.B; Intermittent heart block in athletes. Proceedings of the Sixteenth Congress of Sports Medicine (Hannover 1966), 213.
275. Venerando, A. *Electrocardiography in sports medicine.* Sports Med Phys Fitness 1979, 19: 285.
276. Fenici, R., Caselli, G., Zeppilli, P. et al. *High degree A-V block in 17 well-trained endurance athletes.* In: Sports Cardiology. Lubich, T., Venerado, A. (Eds.). Bologna, Aulo Gaggi 1980, 523-37.
277. Hernandez-Madrid, A., Moro, C., Huerta, E.M. et al. *Third-degree atrioventricular block in an athlete.* J Int Med 1991, 229: 375.
278. Cooper, J.P., Fraser, A.G., Penny, W.J. *Reversibility and benign recurrence of complete heart block in athletes.* Int J Cardiol 1992, 35: 118.
279. Grimby, G., Saltin, B. *Daily running causing Wenckebach heart-block.* Lancet 1964, ii:962.
280. Johnson, R.J., Averill, R.H., Lamb, L.E. *Electrocardiographic findings in 67,375 asymptomatic subjects.* Am J Cardiol 1960, 6: 153.
281. Schneider, J.F., Thomas, H.E., Kregar, B.E. et al. *Newly acquired left bundle branch block. The Framingham Study.* Ann Intern Med 1979, 90: 303.
282. Schneider, J.F., Thomas, H.E., Kregar, B.E. et al. *Newly acquired right bundle branch block. The Framingham Study.* Ann Intern Med 1980, 92: 37.
283. Kregar, B.E., Anderson, K.M., Levy, D. *QRS interval fails to predict coronary disease incidence. The Framingham Study.* Arch Intern Med 1991, 151: 1365.
284. Vasey, C., O'Donnell, J., Morris, S. et al. *Exercise-induced left bundle branch block and its relation to coronary artery disease.* Am J Cardiol 1985, 56: 892.
285. Heinsimer, J.A., Irwin, J.M., Basnight, L. *Influence of underlying coronary artery disease on the natural history and prognosis of exercise-induced left bundle branch block.* Am J Cardiol 1987, 60: 1065.

CHAPTER 10

ITALIAN GUIDELINES
FOR COMPETITIVE ATHLETES WITH ARRHYTHMIAS

A. Biffi[1], F. Furlanello[2], G. Caselli[1], A. Bertoldi[3] and F. Fernando[1].
[1]Sport Science Institute, Department of Medicine,
Italian National Olympic Committee, Rome, Italy,
[2]Scientific Institute H.S., San Raffaele, Milan-Rome, Italy and
[3]Santa Chiara Hospital, Division of Cardiology, Trento, Italy

Introduction

In Italy, participation in a competitive sport is regulated by special national and regional laws concerning preparticipation medical screening. Italian legislation is based on a tradition that limits the free will in situations that could endanger human life. In the last few years, new laws concerning Italian sports have been introduced because of the wide resonance caused by the sudden deaths of some top-level athletes. The most important Italian law concerning the health of athletes stipulates that they must undergo a medical evaluation, including some examinations (resting and Montoye step-test electrocardiogram, spirometry and urine test). Consequently, every athlete without clinical problems must be in possession of a sports eligibility certificate issued by a sports medicine physician. The sports medicine physician is legally responsible for accidents that could occur during an athlete's career and can be charged with medical malpractice (incorrect risk assessment, etc.). Furthermore, the sports medicine physician shares the responsibility with other specialists and consultants, most of whom are cardiologists. The cardiologist is a very important consultant, since lack of eligibility is most commonly due to cardiovascular diseases (50-80%). Therefore, the Italian cardiological guidelines for sports activity make physicians indispensable for sports medicine. These guidelines were published in 1989 and 1995 and were based on the opinions of sports medicine authorities, indicated by the five major scientific cardiological and sports medicine Italian societies (the Italian Hospital Cardiologists' Association, the Italian Non-Hospital Cardiologists' Association, the Italian Society of Cardiology, the Italian Society of Sports Cardiology and the Italian Sports Medicine Federation) (1, 2). Although the Italian guidelines took into account the conclusions of the Bethesda Conference (3, 4), some important differences between the two protocols exist. In the USA, athletes can settle disagreements about their physical health while in Italy, the physician has the sole responsibility. Therefore, for the same cardiovascular anomalies, the Italian guidelines are often more restrictive than the US ones (5). The two guidelines agree on some arrhythmic conditions (coronary artery disease, hypertrophic cardiomyopathy, long QT syndrome, myocarditis,

A. Bayés de Luna et al. (eds.), Arrhythmias and Sudden Death in Athletes, 153–160.
© 2000 *Kluwer Academic Publishers. Printed in the Netherlands.*

etc). However, there are important differences concerning other arrhythmias, such as Wolff-Parkinson-White syndrome and ventricular arrhythmias.

Italian protocols consider that high-risk sports, such as car racing, downhill skiing, diving, alpinism, parachuting, etc. can be very dangerous both for athletes and for spectators because of the appearance of symptoms (syncope, presyncope). Furthermore, the physician can grant a certificate of eligibility for sports involving different levels of cardiovascular activity with reference of sports classification (see Chapter 2).

In this chapter, translated sections from the Italian cardiological guidelines for sports eligibility that concern cardiac arrhythmias (2) are presented.

Italian Cardiological Guidelines

The sports medicine physician who grants a certificate of sports eligibility must be aware that cardiac arrhythmias can be benign but that they can also be the first sign of an underlying cardiac disease. The aim of this protocol is to establish medical guidelines for sport practice in athletes with arrhythmias. This evaluation must bear in mind that arrhythmias can provoke:

i) Too high or too low ventricular rates. These tachy- or bradyarrhythmias can be incompatible with sports activity.

ii) Presyncope, syncope and/or sudden cardiac death.

These latter events are more likely to occur in the presence of heart disease. Therefore, a complete cardiological evaluation, even including invasive procedures, is mandatory for assessing arrhythmic risk in athletes. The evaluation of arrhythmias must include:

i) A complete family history about sudden death, Wolff-Parkinson-White syndrome, cardiomyopathy (dilated, hypertrophic, arrhythmogenic right ventricular cardiomyopathy), mitral valve prolapse and long QT syndrome; the presence of symptoms such as palpitations, presyncope, syncope, asthenia, angor, dyspnea, drop of physical performance, etc.; the presence of infectious disease or fever of recent onset; use of drugs with a potentially arrhythmogenic effect.

ii) Instrumental and blood test data concerning the diagnosis and thecause of the arrhythmias.

The arrhythmologic study is carried out at three levels:

i) The first level includes cardiological examination as well as resting and stress (step-test) electrocardiogram (ECG).

ii) The second level includes an echocardiogram, a stress test (bicycle ergometer or treadmill) electrocardiogram and a 24-h electrocardiographic Holter monitoring. This latter exam should include a training session. In certain conditions, thyroid evaluation may be required.

iii) The third level includes all the invasive and noninvasive examinations needed to exclude the presence of an underlying heart disease (head-up tilting-test, signal-averaged ECG, MRI, resting and stress transesophageal pacing, electrophysiologic endocavity study, etc.)

Judgments about sports eligibility must take into account age, type of sport, seniority of the athletes, etc.

Bradyarrythmias

Bradyarrythmias may be frequently observed in well-trained athletes. They are usually caused by increased parasympathetic tone induced by the high level of physical training.

SINUS BRADYARRHYTHMIAS
A resting heart rate <50 bpm, which does not increase >120 bpm after step-testing is not a normal finding in sedentary subjects. A resting heart rate <40 bpm, which does not increase >100 bpm after step testing is not a normal finding in trained subjects. In these latter situations ECG and Holter monitoring are required to verify a normal increase of the sinus rate during exercise and the absence of sinus node pauses >3 sec.

Third level examinations can be indicated in specific cases.

JUNCTIONAL ESCAPE RHYTHMS
Junctional escape rhythms, wandering pacemakers, isorhythmic atrioventricular (AV) dissociation that disappears during hyperventilation and/or step-testing, do not contraindicate sports activity. In other conditions, ECG and Holter monitoring are required.

ATRIOVENTRICULAR BLOCKS
First degree AV block: PR interval >0.20 sec which shortens during hyperventilation and/or step-testing, does not contraindicate sports activity. In other conditions, ECG and Holter monitoring are required.

Second degree AV block Type 1 or Mobitz 1 require the execution of ECG and Holter monitoring. In asymptomatic subjects without heart disease, sports eligibility can be granted if AV conduction is normal during exercise and if Holter monitoring does not show ventricular pauses >3 sec. However, 6-month controls should be reserved for athletes under the age of 15 years and for those over the age of forty, especially if they are not well trained.

Electrophysiologic endocavity study can be required in specific cases.

Third degree AV blocks require electrophysiologic endocavity study. Sports eligibility is not granted in cases of persistent forms of the disease.

BUNDLE-BRANCH BLOCKS
Incomplete right bundle-branch block (QRS <0.12 sec) in the presence of a normal heart does not contraindicate sports activity. Complete right bundle-branch block (QRS >0.12 sec), left anterior hemiblock, intermittent left or right bundle-branch blocks and bifascicular blocks require further examinations (echocardiogram, ECG, Holter monitoring).

Eligibility for sport can be granted in cases of right bundle-branch block and left anterior hemiblock in the absence of heart disease.

For left bundle-branch block and left anterior hemiblock-right bundle-branch block, sports eligibility can be granted only for sports activities with low cardiovascular engagement. For the other sports electrophysiologic endocavity study is required.

ATRIOVENTRICULAR BLOCKS AND BUNDLE BRANCH BLOCKS
For these kinds of cardiac blocks electrophysiologic evaluation is required.*

Tachyarrhythmias

SUPRAVENTRICULAR ECTOPIC BEATS
Isolated supraventricular ectopic beats that do not increase during exercise do not contraindicate sport activity in athletes without structural heart disease. Otherwise, sport eligibility is subject to the results of echocardiogram and ECG Holter monitoring (any association with bradyarrythmias must be excluded).

SUPRAVENTRICULAR TACHYARRHYTHMIAS
Supraventricular tachyarrhythmias** include paroxysmal and persistent forms represented by reentry tachycardias, atrial ectopic tachycardias, atrial flutter and fibrillation. First of all, athletes with supraventricular tachyarrhythmias must undergo echocardiogram and ECG Holter monitoring. Furthermore, if these latter examinations do not show any significant arrhythmias, athletes with palpitations must undergo a transesophageal pacing at rest and during exercise in order to reproduce symptoms.

Paroxysmal Junctional Tachycardias
Paroxysmal junctional tachycardias (AV node reentry tachycardia and AV reentry tachycardia due to concealed accessory pathway) are the most frequent forms of supraventricular tachyarrhythmias in athletes. Sports eligibility can be granted in absence of: i) heart disease; ii) hyperthyroidism and drugs or alcohol use; iii) relationship between supraventricular tachyarrhythmias and exercise; iv) syncope and palpitations with hemodynamic consequences; v) pathological bradyarrythmias.

Persistent Supraventricular Tachyarrhythmias
Persistent supraventricular tachyarrhythmias (Coumel reentry tachycardia and focal atrial tachycardia) generally contraindicate sports activity and can induce a tachycardiomy-

---

*The bradyarrythmias are discussed in detail in Chapter 7, in the section on paraphysiologic arrhythmias. The bradyarrythmias also include the borderline and pathological forms, most of which have an organic origin, sometimes with a difficult diagnosis.

**Supraventricular tachyarrhythmias and atrial fibrillation are the most frequent causes of long lasting episodes of palpitations in athletes, either during effort or at rest. These conditions also occur in elite athletes (6). The causes are supraventricular reentry tachycardia and atrial fibrillation, which may be easy to reinduce by transesophageal atrial pacing at rest, during ergometric testing or by endocavity electrophysiologic testing. The guidelines recommend the use of transesophageal pacing at rest and during exercise, because transesophageal pacing during exercise is more physiologic than electrophysiologic endocavity study. Currently, electrophysiologic endocavity study is preferred to transesophageal pacing when the athlete has to undergo a radiofrequency catheter ablation.

Atrial fibrillation is a rare event in young people but is probably more frequent in young competitive athletes, affecting males in particular.

opathy. For this reason, radiofrequency catheter ablation is highly indicated in these persistent forms of supraventricular tachyarrhythmias and usually produces good results.

Paroxysmal Atrial Flutter and Fibrillation

These arrhythmias, mainly if prolonged >30 sec, require echocardiogram and ECG Holter monitoring. Transesophageal pacing or electrophysiologic endocavity study can be useful in reproducing the arrhythmias or symptoms and their relation with exercise. Sports eligibility can be granted in absence of: i) heart disease; ii) hyperthyroidism and drug or alcohol use; iii) relationship between arrhythmias and exercise; iv) syncope and palpitations with hemodynamic effects; v) bradyarrythmias.

Chronic Atrial Flutter and Fibrillation

These arrhythmias contraindicate sports activity.

Chronic atrial fibrillation can be compatible with sports activities with a low cardiovascular engagement (group B2) in the absence of: i) structural heart disease; ii) symptoms; iii) a ventricular rate <200 bpm during exercise; iv) bradyarrhythmias (heart rate <40 bpm and ventricular pauses >3000 msec); Wolff-Parkinson-White syndrome.

VENTRICULAR PREEXCITATION

Wolff-Parkinson-White Syndrome

Wolff-Parkinson-White syndrome has a prevalence of 1.5% in the young population and generally shows the following arrhythmias: i) AV reentry tachycardia. Usually, this arrhythmia utilizes a reentry circuit, which involves the AV node conduction in an anterograde way and the accessory pathway in a retrograde way (orthodromic tachycardia). The form utilizing the accessory pathway in an anterograde way is less common (antidromic tachycardia). ii) Atrial fibrillation can be present in a preexcited form or not and it can worsen in ventricular fibrillation.

Wolff-Parkinson-White syndrome requires echocardiogram and ECG Holter monitoring to disclose an underlying heart disease and to identify clinical arrhythmias. However, transesophageal pacing at rest and during exercise is mandatory for symptomatic and asymptomatic athletes with Wolff-Parkinson-White syndrome who need certification of sports eligibility.

Sports eligibility can be granted in absence of: i) structural heart disease; ii) documented atrial fibrillation and supraventricular tachyarrhythmias >30 sec; iii) relationship between exercise and tachyarrhythmias (even for nonsustained forms <30 sec).

Electrophysiologic Criteria

Athletes with Wolff-Parkinson-White syndrome and two or more of the following criteria are not considered eligible for sports activity: i) induced atrial fibrillation with a shortest R-R interval between preexcited beats ≤240 msec (at rest) and ≤200 msec (during exercise); ii) induced atrial fibrillation lasting >/= 30 sec; iii) high atrial vulnerability (easy induction of atrial fibrillation using a nonaggressive stimulation protocol); iv) induced AV reentry tachycardia.

In athletes with "borderline" electrophysiologic results, mainly if they practice high risk activities (car racing, underwater sports, alpinism, etc.), transesophageal pacing has to be repeated yearly.

Transesophageal pacing has to be repeated every 3 years even in athletes under the age of 15 years and in those over the age of 30 years because of possible spontaneous variations of the electrophysiologic parameters of the accessory pathway.

Short P-R interval
This anomaly does not contraindicate sports activity in asymptomatic athletes, in the absence of heart disease. In symptomatic subjects see sections on supraventricular tachyarrhythmias and ventricular preexcitation.

VENTRICULAR ECTOPIC BEATS
Ventricular ectopic beats* require the following examinations: i) echocardiogram for finding heart disease (arrhythmogenic right ventricular dysplasia, dilated, ischemic and hypertrophic cardiomyopathy, mitral valve prolapse, myocarditis, congenital and valvular heart disease, etc.; and ii) ECG Holter monitoring.

Sports eligibility can be granted in the absence of: i) underlying heart disease; ii)R/T phenomenon, frequent ventricular couplets and triplets with R'-R' <400 msec, ventricular tachycardia >120 bpm; iii) relationship between exercise and arrhythmia.

In the absence of heart disease but in the presence of electrophysiologic findings which suggest that the individual is at risk, athletes have to be reevaluated after 4 months of detraining. Otherwise, signal averaged ECG, electrophysiologic study and cardiac magnetic resonance imaging are mandatory. Individual athletes with aborted sudden death can return to sports activity if the cardiac substrate responsible for the malignant arrhythmia is no longer present (myocarditis with VT/VF, commotio cordis and Wolff-Parkinson-White syndrome after catheter ablation of the accessory pathway).

SLOW VENTRICULAR TACHYCARDIA
Slow ventricular tachycardia (heart rate <120 bpm) does not contraindicate sports activity in the absence of heart disease. However, this kind of ventricular tachycardia requires echocardiogram, ECG and Holter monitoring to verify the overdrive suppression of the arrhythmia during exercise and the absence of an underlying heart disease. Furthermore, cardiological evaluations every 6 months are needed

FASCICULAR AND ITERATIVE VENTRICULAR TACHYCARDIA
Fascicular and iterative ventricular tachycardia arrhythmias require third level arrhythmological study. Sports eligibility may be individually granted.

---

*Ventricular arrhythmias and, in particular, complex ventricular ectopic beats and sustained or nonsustained ventricular tachycardia are often a problem for the sports medicine physician. In fact, there are some life-threatening ventricular arrhythmias that can occur in previously asymptomatic athletes, without the documentation of any arrhythmologic substrate (early phase of arrhythmogenic right ventricular dysplasia, dilated cardiomyopathy, hypertrophic cardiomyopathy, idiopathic VT/VF, Brugada syndrome, etc.) (7) (see Chapter 7).

MALIGNANT VENTRICULAR TACHYARRHYTHMIAS
Sustained ventricular tachyarrhythmia, torsade de pointes, ventricular fibrillation and cardiac arrest contraindicate sports activity.

In some cases, third level arrhythmologic study may exclude the possibility of a recurrence of the arrhythmia. Only in these latter cases can sport eligibility be reconsidered.

LONG QT SYNDROME
Long QT syndrome contraindicates sports activity, even in absence of documented ventricular tachyarrhythmias.

Appendix

PACEMAKER AND IMPLANTABLE CARDIOVERTER DEFIBRILLATOR
Patients with third degree AV block or sick sinus syndrome that has been completely corrected by pacemaker implantation (in particular with rate-responsive options), can practice recreational sports (Group A) as well as sports with low cardiovascular engagement (Group B2). Sports should not damage the functioning of the device.

Sports eligibility cannot be granted to patients with an implantable cardioverter defibrillator.

ATHLETES WHO HAVE UNDERGONE A SURGICAL OR RADIOFREQUENCY CATHETER ABLATION
Athletes who have successfully undergone a catheter radiofrequency or surgical ablation of the accessory pathway (Wolff-Parkinson-White syndrome) or of another arrhythmogenic substrate can be considered eligible for sports activity if: i) they do not show the presence of an underlying heart disease; ii) 4 months have passed from the time of ablation; iii) they are asymptomatic; iv) transesophageal pacing and/or electrophysiologic endocavity study do not induce tachyarrhythmias; v) AV conduction is normal.*

References

1. Comitato Organizzativo Cardiologico per l'Idoneità allo Sport (COCIS). *Protocolli cardiologici per il giudizio di idoneità allo sport agonistico.* G Ital Cardiol 1989, 19: 250-4.
2. Comitato Organizzativo Cardiologico per l'Idoneità allo Sport (COCIS). *Protocolli cardiologici per il giudizio di idoneità allo sport agonistico.* G Ital Cardiol 1996, 26: 949-83.
3. *Cardiovascular abnormalities in the athlete: Recommendations regarding eligibility for competition.* 16th Bethesda Conference. J Am Coll Cardiol 1985, 6: 1166-98.
4. Maron, B.J., Mitchell, J.. *Recommendations for determining eligibility for competition in athletes with cardiovascular abnormalities.* 26th Bethesda Conference. J Am Coll Cardiol 1994, 24: 846-99.
5. Furlanello F. *Problemi cardiovascolari nell'atleta: Ruolo del cardiologo dello sport.* In: Atti VII

---

*A common opinion is that athletes with symptomatic arrhythmias are better treated with radiofrequency catheter ablation rather than with antiarrhythmic drugs. In fact, long-term pharmacological treatment might impair athletic performance and it may sometimes be included in the illicit drugs list.

Congresso Nazionale della Società Italiana di Cardiologia dello Sport. Trento 20-22 October, 1995. Ed. C.E.S.I.: Rome 1995; 31-2

6.   Furlanello, F., Bertoldi, A., Dallago, M., et al. *Atrial fibrillation in elite athletes.* J Cardiovasc Electrophysiol 1998, 9 (Suppl.), S63-8.

7.   Corrado, D., Thiene, G., Nava, A. *Sudden death in competitive athletes: Clinicopathologic correlations in 22 cases.* Am J Med 1990, 89: 588-96.

For further reading, see references in Chapter 7.

INDEX

Developments in Cardiovascular Medicine

Developments in Cardiovascular Medicine

Developments in Cardiovascular Medicine

Developments in Cardiovascular Medicine

Previous volumes are still available

KLUWER ACADEMIC PUBLISHERS – DORDRECHT / BOSTON / LONDON